Epilepsy
SIMPLIFIED

John Paul Leach MD

Rebecca O'Dwyer MD

tfm Publishing Limited, Castle Hill Barns, Harley, Nr Shrewsbury, SY5 6LX, UK. Tel: +44 (0)1952 510061; Fax: +44 (0)1952 510192 E-mail: nikki@tfmpublishing.com; Web site: www.tfmpublishing.com

Design & Typesetting: Nikki Bramhill BSc Hons Dip Law
First Edition: January © 2011

ISBN: 978 1 903378 73 1

Printed by Gutenberg Press Ltd., Gudja Road, Tarxien, PLA 19, Malta. Tel: +356 21897037; Fax: +356 21800069.

Contents

Preface

I realise that giving a book a title with the word 'simple' gives our so-called friends an easy laugh, but I think that simplicity is an under-rated virtue. All too often, experts are keen to show how difficult their area of interest can be; a kind interpretation would be that they just want to engage the reader's intellectual curiosity, a less kind one that they are trying to show how only someone as smart as them could untangle such difficult knotty problems. They work hard at giving their subject an exclusive air, which is great if you're selling handbags, but not so good if you are trying to stimulate and educate.

Epilepsy is a common condition, and it is important that all health professionals have a working knowledge of how epilepsy interacts with their own area of expertise. Limited exposure to the condition makes it easy to believe that epilepsy is a mysterious or sinister condition, with all the judgement and stigma that follows from these ancient beliefs. Some grounding in the clinical manifestations leaves the student in no doubt about the range of presentations and treatments.

We would argue that patients with epilepsy are helped in greatest number when knowledge of epilepsy is increased in all health professionals with whom they have to deal. To do this we have to educate psychiatrists, acute physicians, primary care doctors and nurses in how simple steps can make a significant difference to the way the condition is borne and treated.

This book, therefore, is intended to make clear the important concepts of epilepsy cause, prognosis, and treatment available to all. We have included some thought exercises and some common themes to help you understand how we think the condition affects sufferers and their families.

The more astute among you may notice that the book is coauthored by doctors on either side of the Atlantic. In this case we hope you will not be offended if the occasional extra 'U' or passive 'S' disagrees with your own normal practice - if you don't like it - tough. It's not our fault - blame the French.

We hope that doctors, no matter their own specialty, will find something to help in their encounters with patients who have seizures, ensuring that even if patients have seizures, they don't have to suffer from their epilepsy.

Glossary

ABN	Association of British Neurologists
AED	Anti-epileptic drugs
CPS	Complex partial seizures
CT	Computed tomography
DNET	Dysembryoplastic neuroepithelial tumours
EEG	Electro-encephalography
GABA	Gamma-aminobutyric acid - the most widespread inhibitory neurotransmitter
GEFS+	Generalized epilepsy with febrile seizures plus
IGE	Idiopathic generalised epilepsy
ILAE	International League Against Epilepsy - the main grouping of medical professionals interested in the care of patients with epilepsy
LOC	Loss of consciousness
MRI	Magnetic resonance imaging
NCSE	Non-convulsive SE
NEAD	Non-epileptic attack disorder *aka* pseudoseizures
PET	Positron emission tomography

PNES	Psychogenic non-epileptic seizures
PTA	Post-traumatic amnesia
SE	Status epilepticus
SGTCS	Secondary generalised seizures
SMEI	Severe myoclonic epilepsy of infancy
SPECT	Single photon emission tomography
SPS	Simple partial seizures
SUDEP	Sudden death in epilepsy
TLE	Temporal lobe epilepsy

About the authors

John Paul Leach studied medicine in his home town of Glasgow, and after finishing his research thesis on *The New Anti-epileptic Drugs* went to train in neurology and clinical neurophysiology in Liverpool's Walton Centre. He likes socialising and long walks on the beach, oops sorry, wrong summary.... He has been a Consultant Neurologist in Glasgow since 2002, and serves on a number of committees including the UK branch of the ILAE. He is occasionally to be seen speaking at meetings, leaving international delegates with the most puzzled of expressions when they try and untangle bad jokes told in a broad Glasgow accent.

Rebecca O'Dwyer was born and grew up in Dublin, Ireland, before moving and graduating from the University of Munich. There she studied epilepsy under Professor Soheyl Noachtar for her doctoral thesis. She was one of the recipients of the Young Investigator's Award at the 2005 International Epilepsy Congress for this work. She then completed a three-year epilepsy research fellowship at the Cleveland Clinic Epilepsy Centre, during which she won the Young Investigator's Award at the International Heart-Brain Summit in 2008 and the Thomas Epilepsy Award in 2009. She has authored many articles and presented her work at many national and international conferences. Currently she is pursuing her clinical neurology training at Georgetown University Hospital, Washington, D.C., USA.

Acknowledgements

This book could never have come about without the tenacity and enthusiasm of Jonathan Gregory and Nikki Bramhill at TFM publishing - I thank them profusely. Thanks are also due to Professor Donald Hadley, Dr Aslam Siddiqui, and Dr Veronica Leach from the departments of Neuroradiology and Neurophysiology at the Southern General Hospital for their technical help in interpreting the images in the investigations section. Dr Graeme Sills helped make sure I was not too wide of the mark when it came to basic science, and Professor Mike Kerr supervised my grasp of epilepsy in patients with learning difficulty. And of course thanks to Becky for her vision and persistence during otherwise trying times.

It is shameful that thanks are easier given in print than in person: I will, however, always be grateful to the teachers, colleagues, mentors, and friends who have made this kind of venture possible - Martin Brodie, David Chadwick, Phil Smith, Dave Smith, Graeme Sills, and Mike Kerr have all fulfilled multiple roles. This venture is far more modest than their own achievements, but it would never have happened without their teaching, inspiration, and morale boosting.

This bit is an ideal opportunity to acknowledge the support given by my long-suffering wife and not-so-long-suffering children. This book has given them some respite from my ill-tempered rants (what passes for social comment in our house), embarrassing dress sense, and highly suspect personal hygiene. They will be disappointed at its completion. And finally to my parents - for as long as I can remember, you've been on my side. No one could have asked for more.

John Paul Leach MD

Firstly, I would like to thank my co-author and mentor, John Paul. I couldn't have had a more enthusiastic or patient mentor while working on this book. He makes writing and reading a textbook fun! I would also like to thank my husband, Srinivas, who never complains when I retreat to my stack of papers and post-it notes, and then fall asleep over them! My passion for epilepsy stems from my mentor Sohely Noachtar, and the original work I did with him, has moulded the direction of my life since. Last but not least, I want to thank my parents, Michael and Patricia, for their continuing support that allowed me to follow my dreams.

Rebecca O'Dwyer MD

Thought for the book

You may wonder why people become interested in helping patients with epilepsy, and why the occurrence of occasional seizures may have such a devastating effect on patients' lives. To clarify this in your mind, it may help to have a think about the following questions before you continue with the book.

Imagine that life stops for you at the moment:

◆ how you would feel if you didn't make it back to your house or back to your room from where you are now?
◆ how would you feel if there had been an episode last week where you had lost time and had to be taken to the local casualty department?
◆ how would you feel if this had happened at work, your colleagues having seen you collapse and injure your face?
◆ how would you feel if you had been told that this was likely to happen again?
◆ how scared would you be about more serious injury happening next time?
◆ how would you feel if someone had said you turned blue and they had to put something in your mouth to stop you swallowing your tongue and choking?

The fear, loss of control, embarrassment, would be enough after a single episode. How much greater would it be if the same things had happened at regular intervals over the last 6 months despite treatment.

◆ how would you feel if you had to take drugs twice a day?
◆ how would you feel if your tiredness, low mood, dizziness, were all possibly attributed to these drugs?

First aid for seizures

I make no apologies for putting this bit in first. The very fact that you are reading this book means that you are in a position to come across someone having a seizure. If this first aid section was buried away, when faced with someone having a generalised tonic-clonic seizure, instead of wondering how to best deal with this, you'd find yourself pondering the pharmacokinetics of phenobarbitone, or the annual risk of recurrence of seizures in an 82-year old woman with two previous strokes. How much good would that do you? Or the patient having the seizure? So here goes....

First aid for someone having a seizure:

◆ most seizures will not require specific drug administration;
◆ don't put anything in the patient's mouth;
◆ protect the patient from injuring themselves. Clear or avoid any situations (e.g. heights) or objects (e.g. traffic, fires, radiators) that could cause injury during epileptic activity;
◆ don't put anything in the patient's mouth;
◆ ensure the patient has a clear airway - put the patient in the recovery position (or at least lie them partly on their side). This will ensure that the tongue does not obstruct the airway;
◆ ensure the pulse rate and volume are adequate;
◆ don't put anything in the patient's mouth;
◆ an ambulance should be called if:
  - there is no history of epilepsy;
  - any injury has been sustained;
  - seizures recur rapidly;
  - cardiorespiratory function is impaired;
  - seizures have evolved new features;
◆ keep an eye on the patient to ensure their safety as they recover;

◆ once the patient begins to regain awareness, make sure they do not wander into danger;

◆ and finally, even when the patient is awake - don't even think about putting anything in their mouth.

Chapter 1
Definition and epidemiology of epilepsy

What is epilepsy?

Definitions

Epilepsy is a very variable disorder. To help form an image in your mind, it may be helpful to define various seizure manifestations and aspects of the disease. Things might at first seem rather complex when we start by saying that while all patients with epilepsy experience seizures at some point, not all patients with seizures have epilepsy. Bear with us, it'll be less complex than you think!

Epileptic

This is a word which shows that something is caused by or related to epilepsy. Given the stigma, it has become politically incorrect to use it as a single word to describe a patient. Actually while I usually find PC phrases jarring, I completely agree with this - it should go the way of other terms which have evolved a derogatory undertone (e.g. 'mental', 'cretin', 'banker'). The acceptable term is 'patient with epilepsy'.

Epileptic seizure

An epileptic seizure is a clinical manifestation resulting from abnormal and excessive electrical discharges in a set of neurones within the brain.

This may involve alteration of consciousness, alongside motor, sensory, autonomic or psychic events, that can be perceived by the patient or an observer. In other words, seizures cause signs, or symptoms, or both.

Acute symptomatic seizure

Acute symptomatic seizures are an immediate response to any form of brain insult, whether traumatic, systemic, toxic or metabolic in nature. They may be referred to in the literature as a 'provoked seizure' or 'situation-related seizure'. Evidence would suggest that having an acute symptomatic seizure does not lead to an increased risk of future spontaneous seizures.

Unprovoked single seizure

An unprovoked single seizure is any seizure (or cluster of seizures occurring within 24 hours), in a person older than one month of age and in the absence of any precipitating factors or possible responsible clinical condition. After a single event (see section on single seizures later) only around half of patients will have a spontaneous recurrence. There are therefore good prognostic and therapeutic reasons for separating out patients having a single seizure from those with a diagnosis of epilepsy. Unprovoked seizures may result from a static brain injury (e.g. cerebral ischaemia, trauma) or a progressive (not acute) injury (e.g. tumour, degenerative disorder). There is an increased risk of recurrence of a single seizure in patients with an underlying brain injury.

Provoked seizure

A seizure with a specific and isolated cause (e.g. immediate aftermath of a head injury, stroke, alcohol withdrawal).

Epilepsy

Now we get to the easy part. Once there have been two or more unprovoked seizures (see above) then the patient is deemed to have epilepsy. Because the prognosis of recurrence differs in patients who have had febrile seizures and neonatal seizures (<1 month of age), these two groups are excluded from this definition.

Epileptic syndrome

Syndromic diagnosis of epilepsy (see later section) tries to group types of epilepsy according to type of seizures and source of discharges. For example, if the epilepsy arises from the frontal lobes then the epilepsy syndrome is said to be a frontal lobe epilepsy. Discussion will follow later on the classification of epilepsy and seizures (bet you just can't wait!).

Seizure semiology

The symptoms and signs noted directly before, during and directly after a seizure.

Status epilepticus

A single epileptic seizure of longer than 30 minutes or a cluster of epileptic seizures lasting for 30 minutes or longer during which the patient has not regained their baseline level of functioning.

Ictal

Ictal is an adjective describing the period of time during any attack (or for the purpose of this book usually an epileptic seizure), e.g. post-ictal drowsiness, ictal spitting.

Interictal

Interictal is an adjective describing the periods of time in between epileptic seizures.

Epidemiology of epilepsy

Epilepsy is a common disease that occurs worldwide and affects patients of any age. It is estimated that the annual incidence of epilepsy is approximately 80 cases per 100,000 people, with development of chronic epilepsy resulting in a prevalence of around 0.5% (Table 1). The incidence varies with age, the majority of newly diagnosed patients being at the extremes (either under 2 years of age or older than 65 years). Annually, about 20 people per 100,000 will have an isolated seizure. The estimated risk of developing epilepsy over a lifetime (the 'cumulative incidence') ranges from 3 and 5%.

A higher prevalence of epilepsy is seen in underdeveloped areas, especially where cysticercosis is endemic. Similarly, epilepsy is more common in lower socio-economic classes, perhaps due to poorer perinatal care, nutrition and hygiene, in addition to exposure to a greater risk of brain injury and cerebral infection. There is no marked gender preference, but males have a slightly higher risk of being diagnosed with epilepsy.

Within 5 years of onset of seizures, 50-60% of patients will enter a long period of remission on starting treatment, many having long-term control. Up to 30% of patients will eventually develop medically refractory epilepsy despite multiple anticonvulsant medication trials. Given the need for ongoing monitoring and possible trials of further drug combinations, this 30% forms a disproportionately large number of the cohort attending specialist epilepsy clinics.

The standardized mortality rate associated with epilepsy is increased 2-3 times, with an increased mortality often directly linked to seizure frequency and seizure severity. Compared to the general population, patients with epilepsy are more likely to be involved in accidents and suicides. In a small but significant number of patients, seizures can have fatal complications - the so-called sudden unexpected death (SUDEP) -

Table 1 Estimates of epileptic demographics in a population of a million people.

New cases each year (incidence)	
Epilepsy (assume 50-80/100,000/year)	500
Febrile seizures (assume 50/100,000/year)	500
Isolated seizures (assume 29/100,000/year)	200
Established cases of epilepsy (prevalence)	
In remission	15,000
Active (5/1000)	5000

with estimates of one death per 250 people per year with severe and refractory epilepsy.

Conclusions

Epilepsy and seizures are relatively easy to define. Some special cases should be differentiated however. Epilepsy occurs all over the world, affecting all ages (particularly at extremes of age), and is quite common.

Key Summary

◆ Epilepsy is one of the prices we pay for having a responsive and alert central nervous system.

◆ Epilepsy is a common disease, occurring in all races and beginning at any age.

◆ Ignorance of epilepsy among healthcare professionals is all too common.

◆ Definitions of specific epilepsy situations can be helpful.

◆ Some seizures only occur in specific provocation - these patients may not have epilepsy?

◆ If you're confused at this stage - don't worry. All will become clear.

References

1. Hauser WA, Annegers J, Elveback L. Prevalence of epilepsy in Rochester Minnesota 1940-1980. *Epilepsia* 1991; 32: 429-45.
2. Annegers JF, Hauser WA, Elveback L. Secular trends and birth cohort effects in unprovoked seizures in Rochester Minnesota 1935-1984. *Epilepsia* 1995; 36: 575-9.
3. Forsgren L, Bucht G, Eriksson S, Bergmark L. Incidence and clinical characteristics of unprovoked seizures in adults; a prospective population-based study. *Epilepsia* 1996; 37: 224-9.
4. MacDonald BK, Cockerell OC, Sander JWAS, Shorvon SD. The incidence and lifetime prevalence of neurological disorders in a prospective community-based study in the UK. *Brain* 2000; 123: 665-76.

Chapter 2
Aetiology and pathophysiology of epilepsy

It should be realised that a seizure is not a diagnosis in itself but a symptom (and / or a sign) of an underlying neurological problem. In many patients, limitations of current investigations ensure that the exact causative process will remain unknown. Although there may be identifiable triggers (see below), it is as important to the patient to explain, if at all possible, why they have developed epilepsy.

Another important clinical factor that should be considered, is whether the seizure was provoked or not, as this may affect the direction the evaluation will take and what, if any, treatment options will be considered.

Aetiology

It is important to evaluate the patient to obtain an idea of any risk factors that might elucidate the underlying aetiology. With the advancement of modern molecular biology and neuro-imaging, fewer cases of epilepsy remain truly cryptogenic. A reasonable history will outline the presence of any of the main causes of epilepsy (Tables 1 and 2).

Febrile convulsions

These seizures are common, resulting from the brain's response to rapid and severe pyrexia. Two to 10% of children with a history of febrile seizures will develop epilepsy later in life, in comparison to 0.5% of

Table 1 Questions to ask: Why should this patient have epilepsy?

Genetics	Family history of faints, fits, drop attacks, or seizures *Also picks up on cardiac problems*
Birth injury	Were you premature, a 'blue baby', or born by emergency Caesarean section?
Congenital problems	Did you walk and talk at the correct stage when you were young?
Febrile convulsions	Did you ever have any fever fits or febrile convulsions when you were a young child?
Head injury	Have you ever had any skull fractures or knocked yourself out for minutes or been concussed for hours?
Infections	Ever had any meningitis or encephalitis?
Brain insult	Have any history of strokes or TIAs?
Alcohol	Regularly drink? How many units per week?
Drugs	Have any history of exposure to street drugs?

children with no history. Around a third of these seizures are prolonged (known as 'complex') and are more likely to effect changes in the brain which may predispose to further seizures. The structural marker for this is hippocampal sclerosis, the most common underlying pathology among patients with temporal lobe epilepsy. Some genetic conditions may make development of this pathology more likely.

Head trauma

The seminal study by Annegers *et al* looking at the incidence of epilepsy after head injury was reported in 1998. This showed that the more severe the head injury, the more likely epilepsy is to develop (Table 3), and that this risk is highest in the earliest stages. Post-traumatic epilepsy occurs

Table 2 Relative frequency of causes of epilepsy.

Genetic	10-30%
Vascular	10-20%
Congenital malformations	5-10%
Neurodegenerative disorder	5-10%
Hippocampal sclerosis	5-10%
Neoplasm	5-10%
Trauma	5%
Childhood epilepsy syndrome	5%
Toxic / metabolic disorder	5%
Single gene disorder	1-2%
Unknown cause	30%

Table 3 Risk of developing epilepsy after head injury of various severity [1].
Adapted from Annegers J, Hauser AW, Coan SP, Rocca WA. A population-based study of seizures after traumatic brain injuries. N Engl J Med 1998; 338: 20-4.

	Ratio of risk increase (95% CI)			
	Year 1	**Year 1-4**	**Year 5-9**	**>10 years**
Mild head injury (<30 mins LOC or PTA)	3.1 (1.0-7.2)	2.1 (1.1-3.8)	0.9 (0.3-2.1)	1.1 (0.5-2.1)
Moderate head injury (LOC 30 mins to 24 hours, or a skull fracture)	6.7 (2.4-14.1)	3.1 (1.4-6.0)	3.1 (1.2-6.2)	1.8 (0.8-3.6)
Severe head injury (LOC or PTA >24 hours, subdural haematoma, or brain contusion)	95.0 (58.4-151.2)	16.7 (8.4-32.0)	12.0 (4.5-26.6)	4.0 (1.1-10.2)

LOC = loss of consciousness; PTA = post-traumatic amnesia

much more frequently with open head trauma (where there is an accompanying skull fracture), and the risk is greatest if damage occurs in large areas or involves frontal and temporal lobes, with 50-60% of patients experiencing their first (late) seizure within the first 12 months after injury. Dural breach, encephalomalacia, intracranial haematoma and prolonged post-traumatic amnesia have all been found to increase the risk of developing epilepsy. Severe head injury will give an increase in risk of developing epilepsy that remains significantly higher even a decade later.

Family history

A rudimentary family history will bring out any genetic predisposition for epilepsy. This usually only applies to those with affected first-degree relatives, with a two- to three-fold increase in the risk of developing epilepsy where siblings or children are affected.

Developmental delay

Epilepsy and learning difficulty may be the common product of a cortical problem such as cortical dysplasia or ischaemic damage. In a paediatric study, developmental delay or mental retardation was present in 37% of patients.

Some rare metabolic disorders may cause both developmental delay and epilepsy. Examples include Gaucher disease, Niemann-Pick disease type C, various lysosomal and peroxisomal disorders, porphyria, pyridoxone deficiency and Wilson's disease.

CNS infections

Chronic epilepsy is seven times more prevalent among people following meningitis or encephalitis than the general population. Viral meningitis is not significantly associated with epilepsy, which will become more common where there is some cortical inflammation. Table 4 lists the most common CNS infections (and their causative agents), which are associated with an increased risk for epilepsy.

Table 4 Infective causes of epilepsy.

Disease	Common infective agents
Meningitis	*Streptococcus pneumoniae* *Neisseria meningitides* *Haemophilus influenzae* Type b
Encephalitis	**Viral:** *Herpes simplex* Type 1, 2 & 6* Cytomegalovirus*, Ebstein-Barr virus, Varicella* Measles*, Mumps, Rubella* Arboviruses HIV Enterovirus JC Virus* **Bacterial: (uncommon)** *Borrelia burgdorferi* *Brucella* spp. *Mycobacterium tuberculosis* *Mycoplasma pneumoniae* *Rickettsia rickettsii* *Treponema pallidum* **Protozoal*: (uncommon)** Amoebic meningoencephalitis* Toxoplasmosis **Fungal*: (uncommon)** *Cryptococcus neoformans* Coccidioidomycosis Blastomycosis Histoplasmosis Aspergillus *Candida*
Cerebral malaria	*Plasmodium falciparum*
Pyogenic cerebral abscess	*Streptococci* spp. *Bacteroides* Gram negative bacilli *Clostridia* spp. *Actinomyces* *Nocardia*
Neurocysticerosis	*Taenia solium*
Tuberculoma	*Mycobacterium tuberculosis*

* denotes infective agents more commonly found among immunocompromised patients.

Cerebrovascular disease

Cerebrovasular disorders may cause gliosis and scarring which will lead to a predisposition to seizures. Table 5 illustrates a brief overview of the risk arising from specific vascular problems.

Table 5 Risk of developing epilepsy in relation to cerebrovascular disease.

Cerebrovascular disease	Increased risk for epilepsy
Cerebral haemorrhage	
Within first week	30%
Subarachnoid haemorrhage	20-34%
Overall	5-10%
Cerebral infarction	
Within 12 months	6%
Within 5 years	11%
Occult degenerative cerebrovascular disease	5-10%
Arteriovenous malformations	
Age: 10-19 years	44%
20-29 years	31%
30-60 years	6%
Cavernous haemangioma	40-70%
Venous malformations	n.s.
Vasculitides	25%
e.g. Systemic lupus erythematosus	

CNS tumours

Neoplasia will disrupt normal neurological function and may lead to seizures. Different primary CNS tumours have different predispositions to epilepsy (Table 6), but seizures are seen in approximately 50% of all brain tumour patients. Metastases from other primary tumours are also a source of epileptic foci and should also be considered. Conversely, although concern about the possibility of a tumour remains common, only around 5% of all newly diagnosed cases of epilepsy are associated with CNS neoplasms.

Table 6 Risk of epilepsy with specific neoplasms.

CNS tumour	Percentage of patients experiencing epilepsy
Glioma	
Oligodendrogliomas	92%
Astrocytomas	70%
Glioblastomas	37%
Ganglioma	80-90%
Dysembryoplastic neuroepithelial tumour	Circa 100%
Hypothalamic hamartoma	Circa 100%
Meningioma	20-50%

Primary diseases associated with epilepsy

Neurocutaneous disorders

This term covers a number of genetic disorders with cutaneous and neurological effects. They will usually be uncovered by physical examination, but may be hinted at by a family history.

Tuberous sclerosis

Tuberous sclerosis is inherited in an autosomal dominant fashion and is caused by mutations in the *TSC1* or *TSC2* genes. This condition leads to a form of cortical dysplasia, with epilepsy being the presenting symptom in over 80% of all patients, either occurring in the neonatal period as West or Lennox-Gastaut syndrome, or later as adult onset partial or generalized epilepsy.

Neurofibromatosis type 1

Neurofibromatosis is also inherited dominantly with practically complete penetrance, but around half of the presented cases are due to spontaneous mutations. The incidence of epilepsy in these patients is 5-10%, taking various forms and presenting at any age.

Sturge-Weber syndrome

Sturge-Weber syndrome causes unilateral or bilateral port wine naevus, epilepsy, hemiparesis, mental impairment and ocular signs. Epilepsy is a common first symptom and at least 70% of patients develop epilepsy by their fourth birthday.

Other chromosomal disorders

Other chromosomal disorders such as Down's syndrome, Fragile X syndrome and Ring chromosome 20 will be associated with both systemic signs and epilepsy - the latter being of uncertain mechanism. In some genetic disorders, focal cortical changes can become apparent with investigation, such as lissencephaly, anencephaly, agyria, agenesis of the corpus callosum and periventricular nodular heterotopia.

Pathophysiology of epilepsy

Whatever the underlying pathology, the abnormality at the heart of seizures is apparently spontaneous sustained repetitive firing of neurones. This may at times be synchronised, and it may either spread widely (generalise) or remain in a specific area of the cortex. It may reasonably be asked why neurones should spontaneously do this.

Disturbance of normal cortical structure (scarring, increase in glial cells) will have important effects. The gliotic tissue will not be as able to

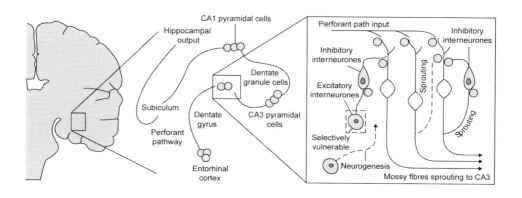

Figure 1 A schematical representation of the pathophysiology of hippocampal sclerosis [3]. *Reproduced with permission from Chang B, Lowenstein D. Mechanisms of disease epilepsy. N Engl J Med 2003; 349: 1257-66. Copyright © 2003 Massachusetts Medical Society. All rights reserved.*

maintain the biochemical environment, and such instability (excessive stimulation or reduced inhibition) leads to changes in cell connectivity and structure, each leading to further instability and a tendency for more epileptogenesis. The histological changes around hippocampal sclerosis provide some evidence of a cascade of abnormalities. As a result of the damage done by febrile convulsive activity, cells in the dentate gyrus which are more able to become involved in neurogenesis form new connections and circuits (so-called mossy fibre sprouting), which are recurrent and excitatory. Excitatory cells which should usually stimulate inhibitory neurones may be more prone to this damage, meaning that the brain will fail to produce enough negative feedback to episodic excitation.

There are probably neurochemical changes which produce some seizures, with studies suggesting that there is a lack of effect of inhibitory systems (usually involving gamma-amino butyric acid) or an excessive effect of excitatory systems (usually involving glutamate or aspartate. Such net changes may come about because of changes in chemical concentration or altered receptor sensitivity or receptor number.

Conclusions

Almost anything that affects the brain can cause seizures. A reasonable history should uncover these. Many patients will, however, report no risk factors. Studies have shown a large number of ways to induce seizure activity in animal models. We remain uncertain, however, about the relative contributions of these in our patients.

Key Summary

◆ There are a great many causes of epilepsy.

◆ Anything which causes focal damage to the cerebral cortex may precipitate immediate or delayed seizures.

◆ Any systemic condition which changes neuronal excitability may cause immediate excitability.

◆ Seizures consist of sustained synchronised neuronal discharges causing symptoms or signs.

◆ The basic processes underlying seizures and epilepsy are not completely elucidated: they depend on networks where excitation is enhanced or inhibition is reduced.

References

1. Annegers J, Hauser AW, Coan SP, Rocca WA. A population-based study of seizures after traumatic brain injuries. *N Engl J Med* 1998; 338: 20-4.
2. Hauser WA. Epidemiology of epilepsy in children. *Neurosurg Clin N Am* 1995; 6(3): 419-29.
3. Chang B, Lowenstein D. Mechanisms of disease epilepsy. *N Engl J Med* 2003; 349: 1257-66.
4. Hauser WA, Annegers J, Elveback L Prevalence of epilepsy in Rochester Minnesota 1940-1980. *Epilepsia* 1991; 32: 429-45.
5. ForsgrenL, Bucht G, Eriksson S, Bergmark L. Incidence and clinical characterisation of unprovoked seizures in adults: a prospective population-based study. *Epilepsia* 1996; 37: 224-9.
6. Shorvon SD. The aetiology of epilepsy. In: *The Treatment of Epilepsy*. Shorvon SD, Perucca E, Engel J, Eds. Oxford, UK: Wiley Blackwell, 2009.

Chapter 3

General history taking

In neurology, it is often held that the diagnosis is founded 90% on the history obtained. If this is true of neurological disorders (and I think it certainly is!), where there are clinical signs to be found of neurological deficit, then clinical history is even more important in epilepsy, where clinical signs are rare.

The history taking process can be more fraught in dealing with epilepsy, particularly where there is recent onset. Discussed below are the main differentiating points in taking a history on new onset epilepsy (where differential diagnosis is important) compared to that required from established refractory epilepsy (Tables 1-3). We have focused on the most important information that should be provided to all patients with epilepsy. Although patients may have been having seizures for many years, you can never take for granted that someone else has addressed issues of safety or lifestyle. In fact, where the diagnosis is longstanding, it is important to bear in mind that some issues (e.g. fertility, driving, occupational safety) may be changed in their relative importance as patients get older, or as circumstances change.

History of new onset events

These histories are made more challenging by the heightened emotions evident in the patients and the eye witnesses. Reviewing recordings of seizures taken during monitoring, it is easy to see exactly why witnesses

Table 1 History for new events - patient history.

- How many events?

- How many types of events?

- Over what time?

- Any provoking / precipitating factors?

- For each type of event
  - What's the first thing you notice?
  - How long did that go on for?
  - And then what?
  - And then what? etc.

- If you lost awareness, what's the first thing you remember afterwards?

- How long did it take to recover?

- Did you bite your tongue?

- Did you wet yourself?

- Did you have a headache?

- Did you have sore muscles?

are so anxious after witnessing a friend or relative having a generalised seizure. In fact, it might be surprising that levels of anxiety are not higher. It is vital that the patients and, sometimes moreso, the relatives are allowed to express their fears and anxieties, and sometimes this means that the clinician has to let both sides have their say before gathering specific facts. Failure to let them 'blow off steam' may give them the wrong impression that you are not listening to them. If they are to have faith in your treatment and investigative decisions, you have to gain the trust of all sides before you can move on. Letting the patients and carers express

Table 2 History for new events - eye witness history.

- How many have you seen?

- Are they all the same?

- For each type of event
    - What's the first thing that happens?
    - How long did that go on for?

- For each type of event
    - What's the first thing you notice?
    - How long did that go on for?
    - And then what?
    - And then what? etc.

Table 3 For recurrent events / established epilepsy.

- When was diagnosis of epilepsy made?

- By whom?

- What tests were done?

- Were there any abnormalities?

- What treatments have been tried?

- For each one
    - What effect did it have on seizures?
    - What side effects did it have?
    - What was the duration of use / maximum dose?

N.B. If there is any doubt about the nature of the events (or emergent events) then follow the same procedure as for new events themselves also has the added advantage of uncovering any particular anxieties at an early stage. This can help instil trust when these particular fears are addressed in the closing parts of the consultation.

In searching out specific facts, I find it useful to explain clearly what you intend to do; I am explicit that I will be looking for the patient's recall of events, followed by the relative's or eye witness's account, explaining how the diagnosis of events causing loss of consciousness requires a good analysis of both symptoms and signs. I will usually set up that I am looking at three phases: the build up, the attack itself, and the process of recovery. This helps to focus the history taking, and allows for more direct questioning later. If there has been more than one attack, the first tactic is to ascertain how many episodes there have been, over what time and, most crucially, if they have all been the same. If they are all the same, I ask them to speak about the most vivid or recent one. If they are different, I will talk about each type in turn, alternating between patient and eye witness to obtain a separate summary of each type.

Turning firstly to the patient, I would start with an open question: "What do you remember about the event that had you taken to hospital?" - or "What do you remember about the first type of attack?". While open questioning and patient expression are important, do not hesitate to ask about specific features during their description. In fact, while patients will focus on their loss of awareness and resultant fear, you may need to ask specifically about particular prodromal symptoms or auras.

Similarly, eye witnesses will focus on the more dramatic features and need to be asked about, for example, colour change, or eye opening. Nothing should be taken for granted; in particular, the description of movements should not be assumed to be correct. Do not assume that the description of "then she started fitting" is necessarily accurate. The eye witness may need to be offered several alternatives (e.g. tremor, jerking, shivering, twitching, thrashing), often with dignity-threatening demonstration from the clinician! The trick in this setting is to have a clear picture (or video!) in your own mind, often running through the sequence of events as the description continues to ensure you have an accurate list of the order of events.

Other aspects of the history (predisposing factors and other events) may help with the differential diagnosis and, where appropriate, epilepsy classification.

Lastly, the rest of the interview should be devoted to addressing the patient's fears, family anxieties, and looking at the lifestyle implications of the recent event. Fear about harm resulting from the seizure should be uncovered and addressed, and may be partly allayed by an appropriate and realistic clarification of first aid for seizures and the best measures to ensure safety and minimise inconvenience resulting from seizures.

Conclusions

One of the things that can make epilepsy fascinating and frustrating is the constant need to keep evaluating and thinking. As in the book *The Citadel*, the key point is to "take nothing for granted". Events that don't respond to treatment may not be amenable to anti-epileptic drugs - either because they are refractory epilepsy or because they are not epileptic. In making judgements about events that you have not seen, you will inevitably be getting something wrong. Your job is not to always be right, but to reduce the errors and correct them when they become apparent.

Key Summary

◆ A history of epileptic events can be difficult to obtain.

◆ If things don't go to plan, keep on thinking.

◆ Questions for patients should be open, but offering options can be helpful.

References

1. Smith PE, Leach JP. Epilepsy - time for review. *Quarterly Journal of Medicine* 2003; 96: 87-9.
2. Smith D, Defalla BA, Chadwick DW. The misdiagnosis of epilepsy and the management of epilepsy in a specialist clinic. *Quarterly Journal of Medicine* 1999; 92: 15-23.
3. Leach JP. When the antiepileptic drugs are not working. *Practical Neurology* 2009; 9: 27-32.

Chapter 4
Differential diagnosis of epilepsy

At first thought, you might wonder if it shouldn't be easy to diagnose epilepsy. Novels and films contain examples emphasising flailing dramatic movements and foaming at the mouth so theatrical it would seem easy enough for the most casual of observers to be certain about the cause. The problem for the busy clinician, of course, is that other conditions can cause patients to move having lost consciousness.

Some neurologists might argue that the epilepsy clinic is harder than the movement disorder clinic or the MS clinic - in these, the doctor at least has the luxury of directly observing and examining the patient's neurological status at his own leisure. Examination then allows documentation of the salient features and a reasonable diagnosis.

Diagnosis of the paroxysmal disorders - those where there are no abnormalities found or experienced in between attacks - however, requires careful history taking. Epilepsy and migraine are examples of paroxysmal disorders, but since awareness is preserved during a migraine attack, the patient will be able to give a full description (and boy, can migraineurs give a full description!) which helps proper characterisation of the disorder. With any episode involving altered awareness, it is important that the doctor obtains as full a description as possible from any eye witnesses.

There are a number of conditions whose manifestations may mimic seizures (Table 1). This list is not meant to dismay, dishearten, or impress the reader, but to reinforce the importance of due care in history taking.

The implications of the diagnosis of epilepsy (medical and social) and the possible effects of treatment, should ensure that the clinician making the diagnosis is experienced in its pitfalls. Some guidelines suggest that the diagnosis should not be made (or non-emergency treatment initiated) unless the clinician has adequate experience and training in this area.

Where awareness is altered enough to cause incomplete or non-existent histories, there may be little certainty. It is vital that the clinician has

Table 1 Differential diagnosis of epileptic seizures.

- Normal phenomena (e.g. déjà vu, hypnic jerks)

- Behavioural phenomena (e.g. in patients with learning difficulties)

- Syncope (cardiac and vasovagal)

- Panic attacks

- Transient ischaemic phenomena

- Spasms (e.g. multiple sclerosis or other disorders of upper motor neurones)

- Migraine

- Transient global amnesia

- Narcolepsy

- Sleep phenomena
  - Sleep paralysis
  - Periodic limb movements in sleep
  - Parasomnias (REM and non-REM)
  - Sleep apnoea

- Provoked seizures
  - Traumatic
  - Metabolic (e.g. hypoglycaemia, hypocalcaemia, hyponatraemia)

---

the confidence to say that he is uncertain. Far better to remain ambivalent and let the passage of time crystallize events, than to have hasty commencement of anti-epileptic medication with all the attendant potential for adverse events and side effects. Experience in this field has demonstrated that more harm is done by hasty diagnosis which has to be reversed in later years than is caused by a delay in commencing treatment.

"Not all that shakes is epilepsy"

A glance at Table 1 illustrates that not everything causing blackouts is epilepsy. While such a list is helpful, it is important to remember that the three main diagnoses in the first seizure clinic are seizure, syncope, and non-epileptic attacks (or pseudoseizures).

Around half of patients referred with loss of consciousness will be considered to have an epileptic cause, and mislabelled syncope and pseudoseizure underpin the majority of misdiagnosis in the community and in tertiary care (most studies suggesting about 20-25% of cases).

The way to differentiate syncope and seizures has been outlined below with helpful pointers shown in Table 2.

Differentiation of seizure, syncope, and pseudoseizure

Differentiation of syncope, seizure, and pseudoseizure depends entirely on obtaining a history from the patient and any eye witnesses. While the story may be coloured or complicated by the emotion and distress surrounding the loss of control and panic of watching a loved one become unwell, the doctor can cut through the attendant distress by thinking always about splitting each descriptor's story into three phases: the pre-attack phase (situation, symptoms and signs), the attack itself (usually from the eye witness alone), and the recovery phase. I would recommend a discussion (if possible) with both the eye witness and the patient in the room. In the interests of clarity (and relative brevity) I make it clear that I would prefer to get a story first from the patient, then from the eye witness, with attempts to get a clear outline of the timing of each phase. While giving patients and relatives an opportunity to unburden their anxieties

Table 2 Seizure, syncope, and pseudoseizure.

	Seizure	Non-epileptic attack (pseudoseizure)	Syncope
Predisposing factors	• Family history • Birth trauma • Febrile convulsion • Meningitis / Encephalitis • Stroke • Head injury • Alcohol / drug use	• Female gender	• Youth • Family history • Medication (antihypertensives, anticholinergics, dopamine agonists, levodopa) • Cardiac disease
Triggering factors	• Sleep deprivation • Alcohol withdrawal • Stroboscopic lights	• Stress • Upset • Conflict	• Postural change • Medical procedures (witnessed or experienced) • Micturition • Heat • Standing • Neck movement • Exercise (cardiac syncope)
Aura or prodrome	• Positive neurological symptoms of memory (déjà vu), taste / smell, sensation, movement (focal jerking)	• Often reported upset	• Palpitations • Dyspnoea • Distal tingling • Sweaty, clammy, hot sensations
The attack	• Movements • Tonic (stiffening) followed by rhythmic jerking • Automatic movements • Cyanosis	• Similar but also flailing • Thrashing • Side to side head movement • Pelvic thrusting • Prolonged motionless	• Pallor • Stiffening or jerks (usually brief)
Sequelae	• Seizure markers (lateral tongue biting, muscle pain) • Focal neurological deficit • Weakness, dysphasia	• Upset, weepy	• Fatigue

surrounding the attack, the discussion in such a setting can be most useful in stripping the attack down to its individual components. It should be said that estimates of timings by onlookers is notoriously inaccurate (especially where there is emotional involvement). Where the descriptor is unsure, it is usually helpful to offer alternatives (seconds, 2 minutes, 10 minutes, 30 minutes?) to gain some impression, however vague.

Sometimes, the flood of details can seem confusing, until a later review of the phases and estimations of time make an objective assessment of cause much easier. It is not uncommon for me to express uncertainty after a clinic visit, only to feel much more certain as the clinic letter is reviewed and corrected some days later!

Syncope

Syncope is very common (estimates suggest it may affect up to one third of the population) and many readers will have some experience of this. It can be defined as a loss of consciousness caused by a decrease in blood flow to the brain. In youth this is most often due to vasovagal syncope, with a drop in blood pressure due to bradycardia caused by an increase in vagal tone. Other factors may trigger individual events (panic, nausea, fasting, being a medical student in orthopaedic theatre), but it is noted that this tendency will reduce with advancing age. The precipitation by exercise at any age is a 'red flag' sign and should merit at the very least an ECG, possibly with other cardiac investigations to exclude, for example, hypertrophic obstructive cardiomyopathy or prolonged QT syndrome.

The response to decreasing cerebral blood flow is to increase sympathetic tone, so leading to the common presyncopal symptoms of sweating, palpitations, pallor, dyspnoea and feelings of anxiety. As blood flow reduces, the patient may notice visual changes (greying, 'white out', tunnel vision) as retinal blood flow reduces and a sensation of dizziness ('lightheadedness' rather than vertigo).

Loss of awareness due to syncope is usually brief, and there is rapid regaining of function with a residual fatigue. Most patients will report feeling 'washed out' for some time (up to some hours) afterwards.

So called 'seizure markers' are not uncommon in syncope. There is no such thing as a 'gold standard' clinical differentiator of seizure and syncope. Urinary incontinence is common in syncope and cannot be used to differentiate it from seizure. Tongue biting also is known to occur in syncope, although this usually involves the tip of the tongue rather than the sides. Severe tongue injuries are much more common in seizure than syncope. It should be noted that all the manifestations of syncope become more pronounced in situations where the patient is not able to lie flat (e.g. in an aeroplane, support from 'helpful' relatives).

Eye witnesses will usually describe pallor and sweating at the onset of an attack. A rapid silent 'slumping' collapse is usual. Movements are usually brief myoclonic jerks, but provoked or attenuated syncope may cause more prolonged and sustained movements. The eyes are usually closed, but may be described as rolling upwards. Recovery is usually quick, with no focal neurological sequelae.

Diagnosis of syncope at any age should merit an ECG. Once cardiac pathology is excluded, the mainstay of treatment is reassurance that these attacks are not damaging or dangerous. This should be followed by appropriate medication review, and general advice about cessation or measures to cut attacks short. Patients should be told to sit down (or lie down if possible) if attacks come on.

Epileptic seizures

Seizures are less common among the population than syncope. Although they can occur without preceding symptoms, epileptic seizures will have an aura experienced by the patient if there is a focal onset (see below). With repeated events, the patient should notice that such auras are stereotyped since the same cortical regions will tend to be involved in the same order.

Eye witnesses may report focal features at onset (posturing, dysphasia, head turning). If there is a generalised tonic-clonic event, the fall will be described with the body stiff and straight rather than slumping. There may be a cry or shout at this stage, followed by rigidity and sustained jerking, which decreases in frequency and amplitude over a matter of seconds or minutes. Pallor and, with sustained movements, cyanosis may be described.

While the features of individual seizures are discussed later (Table 2), the pattern of events may be helpful in coming to a diagnosis. Epileptic events are usually unprovoked, but some patients may notice specific triggers such as sleep deprivation or stroboscopic lights. Postural triggers and triggers by exercise are suggestive of syncope. A characteristic temporal dispersion of epileptic events may be clustering, where runs of events over hours, days, or weeks, are followed by a longer period free of events.

Whatever the seizure type, recovery of awareness from seizure may leave the patient experiencing headache or disorientation for some time - a more attenuated recovery than would be expected from syncope. Markers of generalised tonic-clonic seizures such as tongue biting and urinary incontinence are unreliable (especially the latter) and should not be allowed to direct the diagnosis on their own.

Non-epileptic attack disorders (or pseudoseizures)

There is a great deal of difficulty achieving consensus about the nomenclature of this common and important disorder. Non-epileptic attack disorder (NEAD) is too broad a term (since it covers almost anything!) and pseudoseizures may imply wilful deception on the part of the patient. (Table 3).

Table 3 Naming non-epileptic attacks.

- Pseudoseizures

- Non-epileptic attacks

- Psychogenic non-epileptic seizures (PNES)

Whatever the term used, approximately 5-10% of referrals to first seizure services will be for events thought to have their origins in psychiatric or psychological disorders. Where attacks are few, the differentiation between syncope and pseudoseizures can be difficult; an emerging pattern of frequent recurrent unprovoked events would be more in keeping with pseudoseizure.

Patients may report feeling anxious or upset at the beginning or end of an attack, and may suggest that the attacks are brought on by such emotions. Awareness may be partly retained by the patient.

Features of the attack itself may be enough to make a diagnosis (Table 2). Movements may be more florid, dramatic, or prone to cause self-injury than seizure movements. Formed vocalisation during an apparent tonic-clonic event is suggestive of pseudoseizure. Distractability may be evident during the attack, as may voluntary movement (e.g. resistance to eye opening).

Eye witnesses may have picked up on a heightened feeling of distress or anxiety, and may unwittingly voice this when they describe the recovery phase as the patient calming down. The occurrence of weeping or panic on recovery is rather characteristic of pseudoseizure.

In summary, the diagnosis of pseudoseizure can be difficult as many features may appear to be similar to seizure activity. There are a few concerns about having this diagnosis at the forefront of clinicians' minds, since over-diagnosis of pseudoseizure may lead to undertreatment of atypical seizures or genuine status epilepticus. Some seizure types may appear to have strong psychological manifestations; frontal seizures, for example, may exhibit prominent features of fear, but will usually not have any provoking features and will often arise from sleep.

On balance, though, making a correct diagnosis avoids exposing patients to iatrogenic harm (even death) in critical care settings.

The most important diagnostic information will come from patient or eye witness history. Where any clinical doubt remains, the clinician should not be rushed into making a diagnosis or hasty commencement of anti-epileptic drug treatment. Occasionally, clarity can be achieved by capturing an event on EEG. Recording a typical event (perhaps using suggestion techniques) on video with simultaneous EEG may define the clinical and electrical nature of the attack. If the patient and eye witness agree that the captured event is typical, and the EEG shows no epileptic discharges, then the diagnosis is secured (to the doctor's and patient's satisfaction) and appropriate psychological management can be planned.

Conclusions

Many things can look like epilepsy, but they can usually be told apart by a good history from patients and eye witnesses. The most important distinction is between faints, fits, and pseudoseizures.

Key Summary

◆ Take nothing for granted.

◆ When someone loses consciousness and moves it may not always be caused by a seizure.

◆ A good history taken from the patient and any eye witnesses should help distinguish seizure from other causes.

◆ Where the clinical picture is not certain - say so. Don't force the diagnosis.

References

1. Lempert T, Bauer M, Schmidt D. Syncope: a videometric analysis of 56 episodes of transient cerebral hypoxia. *Annals of Neurology* 1994; 36: 233-37.
2. McKeon A, Vaughan C, Delanty N. Seizure versus syncope. *Lancet Neurology* 2006; 5: 171-80.

Chapter 5
Classification of epilepsy

Differential diagnosis of seizure can be difficult, but some insight into difficult cases can be achieved by considering the type of epilepsy that may be causing the clinical picture. Classification of the epilepsy syndromes remains difficult, with sub-committees devoting many hours to the syndromic and clinical grouping of these diseases.

Notwithstanding the updates in the last 20 years, the most enduring classification is that published by the ILAE in 1981. This 1981 version is a practical system which is easily understood and easily used in clinical practice. While there may be reasonable criticism that it is simplistic in this age of genetic and neurobiological advances, the system allows us to plan treatment with more accuracy. Until someone develops testing to provide a rapid forecast of the likely response to individual anti-epileptic drugs, this system will be with us. The 1989 update has the advantage of allowing flexibility in incorporating future scientific advances. If the reader is not keen on either of these, he should not worry - as always, there will be another one along soon enough! In keeping with the book's aim of simplicity, we will focus on the 1981 version in our discussion (Table 1).

The 1981 differentiation - generalised versus partial versus unclassified

In epilepsy terms, it is helpful for the clinician to consider whether an epilepsy is generalised or partial. A generalised epilepsy is one where,

Table 1 Seizure classification - ILAE 1981 classification.

Partial seizures

- Simple partial seizures (SPS)
  - No impairment of awareness

- Complex partial seizures (CPS)
  - Immediate impairment of consciousness
  - Aura (SPS) followed by impaired awareness

- Secondary generalised seizures (SGTCS)
  - May have preceding SPS +/or CPS

Generalised seizures

- Absence (*aka* petit mal)
- Myoclonic
- Clonic
- Tonic
- Tonic-clonic
- Atonic

Unclassified seizures

through genetic or developmental causes, there is a widespread tendency throughout the brain to initiate seizure activity.

A partial epilepsy (sometimes known as a localisation-related epilepsy) results from a focal area of epileptic activity in an otherwise normal brain. This may result from environmental causes (trauma, infection, stroke), maldevelopment, or genetic causes. Seizures from a partial epilepsy may spread and become generalised (see below), but the presence of an aura (the symptoms at onset of the seizure) may betray the area responsible for initiating the epileptiform discharge.

The type of seizure experienced will give clues to classification. Other clues may come from the pattern of attacks; purely nocturnal events are more likely to result from partial onset epilepsies arising from frontal lobes, while early morning onset is more likely in idiopathic generalised epilepsies. Marked sensitivity to alcohol use and sleep deprivation is more pronounced in idiopathic generalised syndromes such as juvenile myoclonic epilepsy.

In most series, clinicians assessing clinical classification of new-onset cases will admit to a number (usually 5-10%) where clinical evaluation and investigation has failed to yield a cause. In these cases, further evolution of clinical features may help move the patient from one group to another, but we should not be shy in terming patients' epilepsies as 'unclassified'; it reflects thoughtful uncertainty rather than incompetence.

The 1989 ILAE classification - symptomatic versus cryptogenic versus idiopathic

These terms were used in the 1989 classification and allow more flexibility than in the 1981 system. They require a relearning of the meaning of the words since for most medics the terms 'cryptogenic' and 'idiopathic' are interchangeable. While there are advantages, we should recognise the limitations, since this system would have post-abscess epilepsy in the same grouping as that occurring after encephalitis, which may not be helpful prognostically or pathologically.

The 2010 classification

This new classification (Figure 1 and Table 2) attempts to take the best parts of the previous classification systems. It has separated those with a localised problem and termed these as focal epilepsy. These are grouped by severity: those without impairment of consciousness, those with impairment of consciousness and those becoming secondarily generalised. This eschews the term complex partial seizure. The classification recognises the differing semiologies from differing brain regions, and outlines recognised electroclinical syndromes at differing ages.

The terms denoting aetiological grouping have also changed to avoid medical confusion: the titles include genetic, structural / metabolic, and epilepsy of unknown cause.

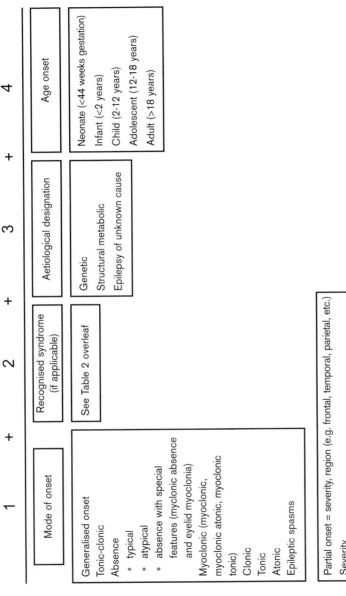

Figure 1 2010 Description of epilepsy and seizures. *From Berg AT, et al. Revised terminology and concepts for organization of seizures and epilepsies: Report of the ILAE Commission on Classification and Terminology, 2005-2009. Epilepsia 2010; 5: 676-85.*

Table 2 Recognised syndromes.

Neonatal

- Benign familial neonatal seizures
- Early myoclonic encephalopathy
- Ohtahara's syndrome

Infancy

- West syndrome
- Benign infantile seizures
- Dravet's syndrome
- Myoclonic encephalopathy in non-progressive disorders

Childhood

- Febrile seizures plus
- Epilepsy with myoclonic astatic seizures
- Benign childhood epilepsy with centrotemporal spikes
- Autosomal dominant nocturnal frontal lobe epilepsy
- Lennox-Gastaut syndrome
- Childhood absence epilepsy
- Epileptic encephalopathy with continuous spike and wave during sleep (CSWS)

Adolescence - adult

- Juvenile absence epilepsy
- Juvenile myoclonic epilepsy
- Progressive myoclonic epilepsy
- Autosomal dominant partial epilepsy with auditory features

Conclusions

The classification of epilepsy is much easier than it may seem at first sight. History, examination and, where appropriate, investigation, will help this in most cases.

Key Summary

◆ Unless you live in 19th century France, don't use 'grand mal' and 'petit mal' as descriptions of seizures or of epilepsy!

◆ Use terms that give cognisance to disease processes underlying the epilepsy.

◆ The classification systems seem complex - but they are actually quite simple.

◆ If you don't like the newest classification system, don't worry. There will be another one along in a minute.

References

1.   Berg AT, *et al*. Report of the Commission on Classification and Terminology: Update and Recommendations. www.ilae-epilepsy.org.

2.   Proposal for revised clinical and EEG classification of epileptic seizures. From the Commission on Classification and Terminology of the International League Against Epilepsy. *Epilepsia* 1981; 22: 489-501.

3.   Proposal for revised classification of epilepsies and epileptic syndromes. Commission on Classification and Terminology of the International League Against Epilepsy. *Epilepsia* 1989; 30: 389-99.

Chapter 6

Seizure types

It is testimony to the enduring powers of the French neurologists of the 19th century that patients and doctors persist in using the terminology devised by Charcot and colleagues in the Saltpetriere. The persistence of the term 'grand mal' and 'petit mal' to describe generalised tonic-clonic seizures and absence seizures, respectively, has been a significant impediment in everyday epilepsy clinics. With the term grand mal being taken to mean 'big seizure', the implication is that everything else is a 'small seizure' or petit mal. Such terminology gives no cognisance of the pathology underlying the seizures, inhibits full description of episodes, and leaves no clue as to the optimal investigation or treatment. I think these terms should be banned, but given the widespread use, we may have to tolerate their use for a while longer!

The ILAE classification (Table 1; Chapter 5) provides a useful way to distinguish between seizure types with some ability to differentiate those from different epilepsy classifications. The different types of seizure are shown in Table 1.

Table 1 Seizure type.

Partial only	15%
Partial and secondarily generalized	60%
Generalized tonic-clonic	20%
Other generalized seizures	5%

Partial seizures

Simple partial seizures

Simple partial seizures can be viewed as seizures where there is a focal discharge contained within a small cortical area. The clinical manifestations depend on the site of the culprit area (the so-called 'epileptogenic zone'). The nature of the initial symptom can help with clinical localisation where these symptoms precede a generalised tonic-clonic seizure. The clinical manifestations of seizures include:

◆ motor manifestations - coming out as positive phenomena such as jerking, spasms, respiratory arrest, or turning;
◆ sensory manifestations - tingling, burning, electric shock, visual changes, rising sensation in abdomen;
◆ autonomic manifestations - skin colour changes, palpitations, pupil dilatation;
◆ psychic or psychological changes - dysphasia, altered memory, cognitive alteration, mood changes, altered perception of size, scale, or distance, or structured stereotyped illusions.

It should be stressed that the distinction between those affecting loss of awareness and those not depends on a reliable eye witness history.

Complex partial seizures

Complex partial seizures may be seen where the discharge spreads to involve the temporal lobe. The initial discharge site may produce a characteristic aura (in fact, a simple partial seizure) before the temporal lobes become involved and awareness is impaired. Such seizures may be associated with automatic behaviour of varying complexity. At their most simple, these will be oral (chewing or lip smacking) or manual (fidgeting, plucking at clothes). At their most complex, these can involve complex behaviours such as wandering, travelling, undressing.

Secondarily generalised seizures

It is always a source of confusion to newcomers when partial epilepsies can cause generalised seizures. In fact, the underlying discharges have spread from a focus to involve both cortices. These seizures would be best known as tonic-clonic seizures; this describes the initial high frequency discharge (leading to tonic muscular contraction) with reducing frequency of discharges leading to jerks of diminishing frequency and amplitude. As with complex partial seizures, patients may report a focal aura signifying the site of origin of their discharges. To the observer, it will be impossible to differentiate secondary generalised seizures from primary generalised seizures (below). Differentiation will become apparent with history of focal onset symptoms, or with knowledge of a pattern of nocturnal events, easy provocation, or focal brain insult.

The clinical features of seizures at various focal points are listed in Tables 2-5.

Table 2 Clinical features of temporal lobe seizures.

- Triple 'A' - aura, absence, automatism

- Slow evolution of seizure

- Auras - visceral, cephalic, gustatory, dysmnestic

- Dystonic posturing of contralateral limb

- Speech arrest (where dominant temporal lobe affected)

- Simple automatisms - oro-alimentary, upper limb

- Autonomic changes (pallor, redness, tachycardia)

- Infrequent secondary generalisation

- Predisposing febrile convulsions

Table 3 Clinical features of frontal lobe seizures.

- Nocturnal generalisation

- Brief stereotyped - rapid onset and offset

- Automatisms - bilateral

- No sequelae

- Frequent secondary generalisation

Table 4 Clinical features of parietal lobe seizures.

- Contralateral sensory symptoms

- Perceptual change - complex illusions

- Auditory hallucinations

- Visual changes, illusions and complex hallucinations

Table 5 Clinical features of occipital lobe seizures.

- Basic hallucinations (lights, shapes) in contralateral field

- Head turning away from lesion

- Perception change (micro or macropsia)

- Eyelid fluttering or nystagmus

Generalised seizures

The different types of generalised seizure are outlined in Table 6.

Table 6 Seizures from generalised epilepsies.

* Absence seizures

* Myoclonic seizures

* Clonic seizures

* Tonic seizures

* Tonic-clonic seizures

* Atonic seizures

Absence

For real epileptologist cool, this name must be pronounced as the French way. These seizures are the ones originally designated 'petit mal' by the French. These episodes are probably among the most common seizure types experienced, but their brevity (a few seconds) and high frequency (often many per day) will lead to misinterpretation of their typical features as being due to laziness or easy distraction, or poor concentration. These short-lived episodes (usually a matter of seconds) are therefore often under-diagnosed, They are different from their focal counterpart (the complex partial seizure) in their lack of automatism, and rapid recovery (often re-taking up activities stopped once the seizure has passed. Absence epilepsy will rarely commence outwith childhood years.

Myoclonic

These are again among the more common seizures, involving one-off episodes of generalised jerks (although predominant in the arms), more notable in the mornings, and are provoked by sleep deprivation or alcohol use. They are usually more pronounced in the arms, and patients may go for some years experiencing these without realising they are of import (in contrast to those who seek medical help for their hypnic jerks!).

Clonic, tonic, tonic-clonic and atonic

Aside from generalised tonic-clonic seizures, the others are relatively rare in adult practice. As a rule the rarer types will occur as part of a group of seizure types in patients with generalised brain disorders causing a more severe symptomatic generalised epilepsy, e.g. Lennox Gastaut syndrome. This group of seizures, by definition, have no focal onset, and their names refer to the movements noted during the seizure.

The tonic-clonic seizure begins with a phase of generally increased tone, causing limbs to straighten and intercostal muscles to contract, thus resulting in exhalation through a partially closed larynx (causing a shout or scream) and jaw closure. After a few seconds, the tonicity becomes rhythmic, causing jerking of limbs, jaw, and respiratory muscles. This clonic phase will usually last a few minutes at most, after which the patient will appear asleep and may be unrousable. On awakening they will be disorientated, vacant, and may report a headache or muscle pains.

Tonic seizures refer to episodes (usually brief) where there is a generalised increase in tone. Clonic refers to episodes (again usually brief) with generalised rhythmic jerking movements, and atonic to those where there will be a generalised loss of tone causing the patient to experience a 'drop attack'. This may sound similar to syncope, but the background of other neurological problems such as learning difficulties, the occurrence of other seizure types, and the lack of provocation should make the distinction easier.

Unclassified seizures

With the best of efforts, there will still be occasions when the origin of seizures is elusive despite good history, imaging and EEG. With all of this information, it remains uncertain whether there is a focal onset to the epileptic events. This is most common when it cannot be determined whether someone has generalised tonic-clonic seizures that are primary or secondarily generalised. In these circumstances, it is important to keep an open mind for future visits (continuing to enquire about other possible seizure types or neurological deficit) and be prepared to carry out further investigation. Treatment will generally be the same as for the generalised epilepsies, utilising the broad-spectrum anti-epileptic drugs.

Clinical differentiation of generalised from partial epilepsies

Table 7 Useful clinical pointers to epilepsy classification in patients presenting with tonic-clonic seizures.

	Generalised epilepsies	Partial epilepsies
Predisposing factors	Family history	Brain injury (vascular, trauma, infective, etc.)
Age of onset	Almost always <25	Any age
Seizure type	No aura	Focal onset ('aura')
Associated seizure type	Myoclonic jerks Absence seizures	Nocturnal generalised tonic-clonic Partial seizures
Investigation	Generalised changes in EEG	Focal change on imaging

When a patient presents with seizures, the nature of the investigation will depend on the clinical assessment of the epilepsy type. The first step is to decide the type of seizure. The next step is to find out if there are other seizure types that the patient has not reported, e.g. myoclonic jerks, nocturnal generalised seizure. When a patient presents with only generalised tonic-clonic seizures, there are a number of useful clinical pointers to epilepsy classification, all of which will help in forming a plan for imaging or EEG (see Table 7).

Conclusions

Unless you have seen the event yourself, you will need a good history to get an idea of the seizures experienced by each patient. These should be named using appropriate terminology. Whenever they come to clinic, the identification of the types of seizure currently experienced should be clarified.

Key Summary

◆ Again - enough with the French terminology - déjà.

◆ There is more to epilepsy than generalised seizures!

◆ When you think about seizures, think about whether the seizure activity will arise from a focal point or is of generalised onset. This will guide investigation and treatment.

References

1. Proposal for revised clinical and EEG classification of epileptic seizures. From the Commission on Classification and Terminology of the International League Against Epilepsy. *Epilepsia* 1981; 22: 489-501.
2. Proposal for revised classification of epilepsies and epileptic syndromes. Commission on Classification and Terminology of the International League Against Epilepsy. *Epilepsia* 1989; 30: 389-99.
3. Shorvon SD. The clinical forms and causes of epilepsy. In: *Handbook of Epilepsy Treatment*, 2nd ed. Shorvon SD, Ed. Oxford, UK: Blackwell Science, 2006.
4. Panayiotopolous CP. *A Clinical Guide to Epileptic Syndromes and their Treatment.* New York, USA: Springer, 2007.

Chapter 7

Diagnosis of epilepsy

History taking

The diagnosis of epilepsy is primarily about getting a good history from the patient. Further investigation will be helpful in characterising any functional and structural changes in the brain, giving you more information about classification, prognosis, and treatment strategies.

The questions that need to be asked differ from setting to setting (Table 1). As always, the main question is whether the ongoing episodes are resulting from epilepsy or not. The only diagnostic test available to you then and there is the history.

For the non-specialist, the wide range of seizure symptoms and signs will make this seem rather daunting. In fact, with adequate time, and a bit of consideration, most doctors (and nurses) will be able to make a good go of it. It is important to lead the patient through the story, getting an estimate of the duration of each stage. The repeated use of the phrase "and then what?..." is a good way of getting patients to volunteer the observed pattern of symptom spread to help you to decide if an attack is epileptic, and, if so, where it originates from. If a specific feature comes out only if it is presented as an option, I would usually document this.

As has been discussed above, epilepsy and its differential diagnosis means awareness is often impaired. This means that the patient's history is not in itself enough, and the account of an eye witness is vital. The same

Table 1 Questions that need to be answered in the epilepsy clinic.

New patient

What are the attacks?

Are they epileptic in origin?

Why should this patient have epilepsy?

Do they need investigation?

Do they need treatment?

What is the outlook?

Return patient or so-called 'known epilepsy'

As per new patient *and*

What treatments have been tried in the past (and why did they fail?)

Is surgery needed?

techniques will elicit the best history from the eye witness - an additional challenge often requiring the doctor to navigate the way through the intense emotion and fear brought about in the onlooker when seeing a relative in distress. Bringing out these emotions may be one of the benefits of attending the clinic.

The importance of ascertaining the dominant hand of each patient should be realised. Where patients are right hand dominant, 90% will have speech centres in the left hemisphere. Where the patient is left handed, there is an even split between the siting of speech centres on the left and right.

For each history, the clinician should be clear about the three phases of the attack:

◆ the onset / the aura;
◆ the attack itself;
◆ residual symptoms (the sequelae).

Patient history

The onset

The patient should be asked about their last memory before the attack. If awake, it may be useful to know how long the amnesia was before attack onset, if there was any situational provocation. The focal nature of any neurological symptoms may direct you to the culprit region (Table 2). While not of focal onset, some patients with generalised epilepsy may experience a cluster of myoclonic jerks at onset of the attack.

Table 2 Focal neurological symptoms - localisation ability.

* Sensory symptoms (opposite parietal lobe)

* Focal jerking (opposite motor strip)

* Visual freezing or freeze-framing (generalised epilepsy)

* Déjà vu (temporal lobe)

* Auditory hallucination (lateral temporal lobe)

* Speech arrest / dysphasia (dominant temporal lobe)

* Abdominal aura (mesial temporal lobe)

* Fear, doom, panic (amygdala)

The attack

In simple partial seizures, awareness will be preserved, but in others, the patient will have a phase of amnesia or loss of contact. This is where the eye witness history becomes most important.

The post-ictal state

The presence or otherwise of headache, myalgia, tongue biting or urinary incontinence can help decide if an episode is epileptic in origin. Limitations of these are discussed above (see the section on differentiating seizures from syncope on p27). Additional information can be gained from the nature of other negative neurological symptoms: dysphasia or aphasia may suggest that the dominant hemisphere has been the source of the discharges.

The eye witness history

The onset

The most important question about this stage is "What was the first thing you noticed?" Eye witnesses may be keen to rush into the description of the movements, but gentle direction in asking about the posture, colour, the eyes (deviated) or whether the patient seemed alarmed, scared, upset, and an estimate of time of each phase will make things much clearer. Clarifying if there has been any head turning or limb posturing may help lateralise seizures to the relevant hemisphere. Once the witness gets used to being asked a sequence of events, they will get into the swing for further stages. If they are resistant to this approach, an explanation of the importance of numerous features in directing investigation and treatment will make them realise how necessary such care is.

The attack

By the time you are eliciting this stage of the history, the eye witness should be used to your tactics. Close attention to the eyes, the colour (red, white or blue), any noises, symmetry (or otherwise) of movement is encouraged. The nature of any fall (slumping or stiff and straight) can help differentiation of syncope from seizure. The eye witness should not (at least not without a fight) be allowed to get away with a description of movement as 'shaking'. Shaking may mean anything from tremor, to twitching, to jerking, to flailing movements, and it should only be accepted (and even then in quotation marks) when the descriptor refuses to accept one of a number of the alternatives (each possibly requiring demonstration by the doctor).

Usually, generalised tonic-clonic seizures involve a short tonic phase followed by clonic movements which will decline in frequency and amplitude over a few minutes. The presence of cyanosis will give useful warning of any danger the patient may be in, and may motivate more aggression in treatment.

It should be remembered that movements in frontal lobe epilepsy may be wild and flailing with an accompanying look of fear and anxiety. These may be difficult in isolation to differentiate from pseudoseizures, but the rapid onset, short duration, lack of reported sequelae, predominance in sleep, and lack of intrusion into life activities (including lower number experienced) may help signal to the clinician that the episodes are epileptic.

The post-ictal state

When the event results from epilepsy, the question "What was he like when the movements stopped?" will elicit a story of a short period of drowsiness, sleep (usually some minutes), followed by a period (again usually minutes) of confusion, distraction, or 'being vacant'.

Diagnostic investigation

Electrocardiogram (ECG)

All patients attending the first seizure clinic or the epilepsy clinic should have at least one ECG. Some studies would suggest that 20% of patients with refractory epilepsy may have a contribution from cardiac problems. Also, cardiac problems such as QT prolongation may be a serious but treatable cause of collapse.

EEG - role in classification

It is a myth long-held by both the medical profession and the general public that electro-encephalography is a useful diagnostic test for epilepsy. In fact, there are few things more likely to cloud an uncertain diagnostic picture than an unwarranted EEG.

Many patients with epilepsy will have a completely normal EEG in between attacks - even those with a recognised generalised syndrome such as juvenile myoclonic epilepsy will only exhibit generalised discharges in around 50% of cases. Conversely, the EEG will be abnormal in a sizeable minority of those who do not have epilepsy, so false positive results will confuse the management of those who have had a routine EEG for diagnostic reasons. In this section we will discuss the EEG, its benefits and potential failings, and ways to enhance its usefulness.

Electro-encephalography is a method of studying cortical electrical activity by application of a number of leads to the scalp. These electrodes are spaced out over the skull, allowing an assessment of where in the brain any activity is greatest. Initially, the patient will have recording done while sitting rested and allowed to become drowsy.

Some activation procedures are carried out whereby the patient is asked to hyperventilate, reducing CO_2 levels and enhancing the tendency for both focal and generalised discharges to appear (Figures 1 and 2).

Photic stimulation will often be carried out, where the patient is asked to look at a stroboscopic light at varying frequencies with eyes open and closed. This will have no effect on focal discharges, but will enhance generalised epileptiform discharges.

As can be seen in Table 3, the EEG is neither a sensitive test, nor a specific one. The role of the routine EEG is in classifying epilepsy, i.e. determining if it is of generalised or partial origin. Since anyone with generalised epilepsy will present at a relatively young age, routine EEG should only be requested in a patient with definite seizures beginning at less than 35 years of age.

Anyone who doubts this should see the confusion and uncertainty caused when a routine EEG throws up some non-specific slow wave

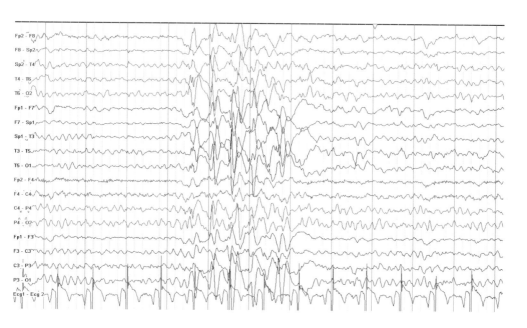

Figure 1 EEG showing generalised epileptic discharges.

a

b

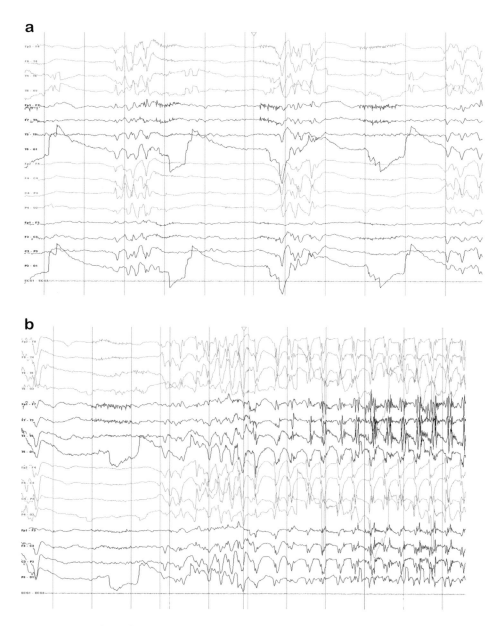

Figure 2 a) EEG showing right-sided focal epileptiform discharges (seen on even numbered leads); b) The same patient as in the top tracing: showing a build up of EEG discharges evolving into a seizure.

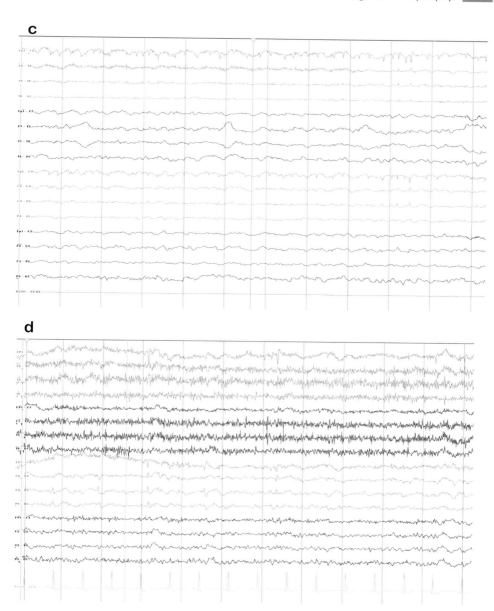

Figure 2 *continued* c) The patient showing some right-sided phase reversals (a sign of focal epileptiform activity); d) Spike and slow waves are seen over the right frontal region (the same patient as in the top tracing).

Table 3 The EEG in different clinical situations.

	Generalised epilepsy	Partial epilepsy	Not epilepsy
Routine EEG	Generalised discharges at approx 3Hz, often with frontal predominance	Focal changes with spikes having most diagnostic usefulness	Usually normal, occasional short-lived focal slow wave changes
	Often normal (circa 50%)	Often normal (circa 70%)	Usually normal (circa 95%)
Sleep-deprived EEG	Enhanced yield of generalised discharges, especially during wakening	Enhanced yield of focal spiking	Usually normal, but some focal sleep-related changes may appear
24-hour EEG	Enhanced yield of generalised discharges, especially during wakening	Longer recordings yielding more abnormalities	Usually normal, but still recognised incidence of asymmetry

changes (or even so-called 'epileptiform abnormalities'!) in a young girl who has clearly fainted. The clinician has, with good intentions, requested an EEG "just to be sure". The return visit then entails a lot of head scratching followed in the worst case by use of an anti-epileptic drug and erroneous application of lifestyle changes. In countries where the health care system means there may be a financial gain for the doctor to request and report the EEG, it can be seen that this incentive may increase use of the EEG.

Increasing the usefulness of the EEG

Where classification or diagnosis of epilepsy is difficult or elusive, the EEG can be helpful. With modification, the EEG's utility can be enhanced by recording an attack. This approach can help distinguish epilepsy from non-epilepsy and also help clarify the exact area of onset, which may be vital information if surgery is to be planned. The following four EEG methods should be considered in these circumstances.

Short video EEG

Differentiation of pseudoseizures from epilepsy can be made easier if a typical attack can be recorded. Suggestion techniques can be used by the supervising doctor or technician to elicit typical clinical features. Use of video recording will allow the patient and eye witness ways to try and record an attack, and can be helpful in demonstrating that throughout this provoked event there are no epileptiform discharges noted.

24-hour EEG

Ambulatory EEG can record continuous EEG activity over 1-2 days at a time. The patient may keep diary accounts of any seizure activity to allow correlation of clinical and electrical events. The period immediately on awakening will be the most likely to produce generalised epileptiform discharges.

Video telemetry

For some patients undergoing consideration of surgery, or for those where they may be unable to keep a reliable diary of their events, admission for video monitoring is justified. These purpose-built suites have camera facilities and the patient remains in the room for the duration of their stay, having the EEG correlated with the clinical status.

Intracranial monitoring

Where there is doubt about the origin of attacks, and where imaging shows either no lesion or multiple lesions, the certainty of origin can be enhanced with placement of intracranial electrodes either in grid form lying across the cortical surface, or depth electrodes with insertion of long tubes into cortical tissue. Obviously, this involves anaesthesia and a small operative risk, so this will only be considered where seizures are frequent enough and severe enough to justify epilepsy surgery, should the results prove conclusive.

Neuro-imaging in epilepsy

Neuro-imaging is central to the evaluation of patients with epilepsy and as advances in imaging techniques are made, we gain more knowledge about the underlying pathology and potential operative options.

The clinical use of X-ray technologies such as computed tomography (CT) has diminished greatly due to the increased superior sensitivity and specificity of magnetic resonance imaging (MRI). The detection of possible epileptic lesions on neuro-imaging can greatly influence and shape the therapeutic strategies chosen by clinicians. Other advances in nuclear medicine, such as positron emission tomography (PET), MR spectroscopy, and single photon emission tomography (SPECT), have some merit as adjunctive imaging modalites, adding clinically useful information, especially in those with no lesion seen in MRI. Thanks to progress in neuro-imaging, the number of patients deemed to have a cryptogenic epilepsy (as defined earlier) will dwindle and the true prevalence of other pathologies will become more evident.

Magnetic resonance imaging (MRI)

Of those patients newly diagnosed with epilepsy, 12-14% will have an identifiable causative lesion on MRI. In contrast, however, 80% of patients with recurrent seizures have structural abnormalities evident on MRI. There are five reasons for doing MRI in patients with epilepsy:

◆ clinically focal onset of seizures;
◆ onset of generalized or unclassified seizures in the first year of life, or in adulthood;
◆ focal deficit on neurological or neuropsychological examination;
◆ failure to obtain seizure control after adequate trial on first line anti-epileptic drugs;
◆ loss of seizure control or change in seizure pattern.

An optimal routine MRI protocol should include T1- and T2-weighted, proton density and fluid attenuated inversion recovery (FLAIR) sequences. These contrasts should be acquired in at least two orthogonal planes, using the thinnest slice thickness possible. A coronal plane gives the best definition of the mesial temporal structures and allows the clearest outline of hippocampal sclerosis.

T1-weighted images (Figure 3) show the grey-white matter junction most clearly and allow the cerebral anatomy to be defined most easily. T2-weighted images are highly sensitive to showing pathological lesions within the cortex. FLAIR imaging (Figure 4) enhances anatomical detail near CSF.

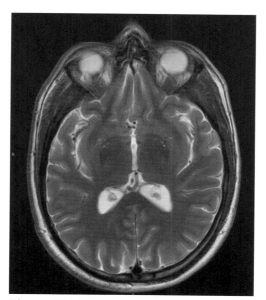

Figure 3 Normal T1 axial image.

Approximately 80% of patients with partial epilepsy have seizures originating in the temporal lobe, the majority arising from the mesial structures of the temporal lobe. The pathological hallmark of mesial temporal lobe epilepsy (TLE) is hippocampal sclerosis which has particular characteristics on MRI. Hippocampal atrophy is best seen on T1-weighted images, while T2-weighted images will show the high signal change. Hippocampal sclerosis will cause other MRI abnormalities such as atrophy of the white and grey matter of the temporal lobe, dilatation of

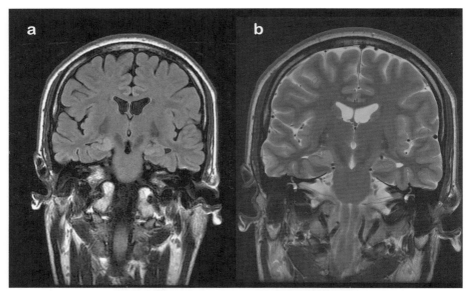

Figure 4 a) Coronal flair MRI. b) Coronal T2 MRI showing a right hippocampal signal change.

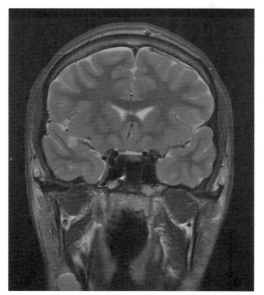

Figure 5 Right temporal lobe lesion on a T1 axial MRI.

the temporal horn and blurring of the grey-white border in the temporal neocortex.

Patients with low-grade primary brain neoplasms often present with focal seizures. The most common pathologies include dysembryoplastic neuroepithelial tumours (DNET), ganglioglioma, gangliocytoma, and piliocytic and fibrillary astrocytoma. In general such lesions are associated with a low signal on T1- and a high signal on T2-weighted images with an absence of vasogenic oedema (Figure 5).

Vascular malformations are another source of focal seizures that can be easily identified by MR imaging. Arteriovenous malformations (AVMs) have demonstrated high blood flow with a nidus, with feeding arteries and draining veins being identified (Figure 6). Cavernous angiomas are small

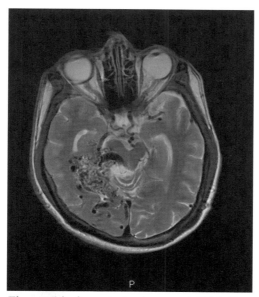

Figure 6 Left posterior temporal AVM. The numerous small flow voids demonstrate a nidus and the larger flow voids are abnormally dilated draining veins. The brainstem is distorted.

dilated veins which have a distinctive appearance on MRI, being circumscribed by a ring of haemosiderin that appears dark on T2-weighted imaging. The central part contains areas of high signal on both T1- and T2-weighted studies (Figure 7).

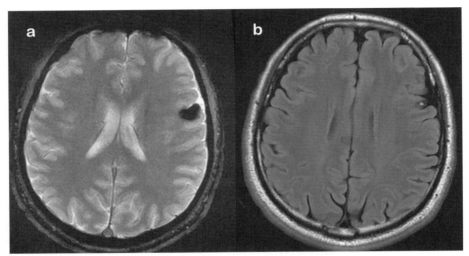

Figure 7 a) Axial T1 and b) axial T2 images showing a cavernous angioma.

Malformations of cortical development pose more difficulties. The important MRI findings of focal cortical dysplasia are focal cortical thickening, simplified gyration, blurring of the grey-white matter junction and T2 prolongation in the underlying white matter, that often forms a cone tapering towards the lateral ventricle.

Single photon emission computed tomography

Single photon emission computed tomography (SPECT) is a useful nuclear medicine technique that measures the regional cerebral blood flow changes in areas affected by epileptic activity. Radioligands are injected intravenously which enter neurones with regional distribution proportionate to the volume of blood flow. Once becoming intracellular, their stabilised forms remain stable *in vitro* for several hours, giving up to 6 hours to acquire imaging. These scans can then be used to assess blood flow during and between seizures. Correct localization of complex partial seizures may be achieved in over 90% of TLE and extratemporal epilepsy patients. The use of subtraction ictal SPECT coregistered to MRI (SISCOM) improves the rate of localization, in particular in cases of malformations of cortical development. SPECT is utilized as a complimentary method for localization of the seizure focus in surgical candidates with intractable epilepsy. It is often of greatest use in patients who have no lesion seen on MRI.

Positron emission tomography

Positron emission tomography (PET) has more technical difficulty than SPECT and is only offered by tertiary care centres. It is another complimentary method that may be used to help confirm or create a hypothesis about the region of seizure onset. Using isotopes attached to glucose and water, PET outlines glucose metabolism in cerebral regions. Cortex responsible for the seizure onset usually shows reduced glucose metabolism and blood flow interictally on PET scans with spatial resolution of ^{18}FDG-PET superior to SPECT.

As MRI evolves with improving sensitivity and resolution, the need for ^{18}FDG-PET may decrease in the coming years.

Conclusions

History taking is an important skill to learn. It forms the basis of the diagnostic process and is less expensive than investigation. Routine EEG should be used with caution. It should only be used for classification in patients with epilepsy, or for prognostication following a single seizure. Specialised methods (ambulatory, video EEG, or EEG with provocation) can help capture an attack and may be more useful in cases of diagnostic doubt or pre-surgical work-up. Imaging is progressing constantly and is usually best with MRI. It continues to be of help in classifying epilepsy, giving patients information about the root cause of their epilepsy, and in pre-surgical work-up.

Key Summary

◆ Again, the challenge is to take a good enough history.

◆ This will tell you if there has been a seizure.

◆ It might tell you if the onset is focal or generalised.

◆ Sometimes it can tell you where the seizure activity has originated from!

◆ How great is that?

◆ Investigation can tell you about brain structure and function.

◆ Investigation can help predict likely classification.

◆ History is still king.

References

1. SIGN 70. Guidelines on diagnosis and treatment of epilepsy. www.sign.ac.uk.
2. ILAE Commission Report. Recommendations for neuroimaging patients with epilepsy. Commission on Neuroimaging of the International League Against Epilepsy. *Epilepsia* 1997; 38: 1255-56.
3. ILAE Commission Report. Commission on diagnostic strategies. Recommendations for functional neuroimaging of persons with epilepsy. Neuroimaging subcommission of the International League Against Epilepsy. *Epilepsia* 2000; 41: 1350-56.

Chapter 8

Anti-epileptic drugs for epilepsy

There has been a recent marked increase in the number of available treatments for epilepsy. For the non-specialist, such profusion may be more bewildering than helpful. I think it is useful to put recent changes in context, allowing a measured response to the additional drugs now at our disposal.

History of AED treatment

The last half of the 19th century saw the first steps made towards pharmacological treatment of epilepsy with the use of bromide salts. Until the discovery of the anticonvulsant properties of barbiturates in 1912, these toxic compounds were the only available anti-epileptic drugs (AEDs). By 1939, Merritt and Putnam had described the laboratory and clinical effects of diphenylhydantoin (phenytoin), a drug with unprecedented activity against partial seizures which remained a first-line AED along with barbiturates, unchallenged for around 30 years.

By the 1960s, a chance discovery led to the discovery of the anticonvulsant properties of sodium valproate: while being used as a soluent for lipophilic calcium channel antagonists, 'control' preparations of valproate were shown to have activity in a wide range of animal seizure models. Carbamazepine, a modified tricyclic agent, was introduced in the late 1960s, and remains a useful treatment for localisation-related epilepsy.

As the 20th century closed, a sustained period of intensive research resulted in the introduction of a number of new anti-epileptic drugs. Vigabatrin and lamotrigine signalled a new era in AED use; the former was the first AED specifically designed to enhance cerebral GABAergic activity, while lamotrigine was later shown to affect sodium channels in their slow inactivated state. Shortly afterwards, gabapentin, topiramate, and another sulphonamide derivative, zonisamide, were utilised in patient studies and given licences for use as anti-epileptics. Drugs such as levetiracetam, pregabalin, zonisamide, rufinamide, eslicarbazepine, and lacosamide were granted licences as the first decade of the 21st century passed, serving to dramatically increase the options available to us in the clinic. In the coming years, it is expected that we will have additional drugs such as retigabine, carisbamate, and brivateracetam to give us more choice in add-on therapy.

On a negative note, the introduction of felbamate in 1995 held a new lesson in caution when descriptions of serious hepatotoxicity and agranulocytosis shortly after a precipitate launch served to severely limit its use.

These are hopeful times: the last 20 years have seen more compounds developed than were discovered in the previous century and a half. As the new century continues, drug treatment of epilepsy has never been so complex or so promising. With even more compounds on the horizon, we may be nearer reaching our goal of maximising both efficacy and tolerability of anti-epileptic drug treatment.

Comparative efficacy of AEDs

The comparative efficacy of AEDs has been hard to establish with certainty. There are many reasons for this, the chief one being the paucity of randomised clinical trials with adequate statistical power to differentiate the AEDs on grounds of efficacy.

Traditionally, most initial trials of AEDs are placebo-controlled studies in patients with refractory epilepsy. Only later, once some anticonvulsant efficacy has been proven, is it considered acceptable to carry out monotherapy studies. Such studies, which are usually carried out for regulatory purposes, are unable to prove significant difference between the compounds, but are simply not large enough to truly determine equivalence. After the Veterans' Administration studies of AED monotherapy run by Mattson *et al*, the number of adequately powered studies comparinig monotherapies was low, at least until the publication of the SANAD studies in 2007. These studies tried to examine the efficacy of AED monotherapy in newly diagnosed patients compared to the respective physician's best choice.

Meta-analysis is one way to circumvent the methodological and ethical difficulties of running large comparative studies of individual randomised placebo-controlled trials, providing a larger cohort for each active treatment. While having its deficiencies, meta-analysis provides a method of extracting data retrospectively from trials. Published meta-analyses have not shown a significant difference between AED treatments.

Recognised anti-epileptic drugs

This section is an alphabetical listing of those compounds which are used, or have been used as AEDs in clinical practice. Tables 1 and 2 provide a short summary. Variations in licensing restrictions may mean that there will be international variations in the scope of use of some of these compounds. Some compounds (e.g. acetazolamide, bromides, progabide) are included for largely historical reasons.

Acetazolamide

By chemically inducing hypercapnia, inhibition of cerebral carbonic anhydrase activity can help to improve seizure control in patients with refractory epilepsy. This is the main action of acetazolamide (interestingly, also a secondary effect of both zonisamide and topiramate). Trials support acetazolamide's use in either localisation-related epilepsy or idiopathic generalised epilepsy. In man, the development of tolerance is unpredictable and may limit its use to intermittent exposure. Dose-related side effects include dizziness, nausea, and paraesthesiae. Other less common side effects include dyspnoea, metabolic acidosis, and renal calculus formation. Animal studies demonstrate this compound's teratogenicity which, alongside case reports of adverse effects in pregnancy, would make this drug unsuitable for use in pregnancy.

Table 1 The established anti-epileptic drugs.

	Spectrum of action	Adverse events — Acute dose-related	Acute idiosyncratic	Chronic toxicity	Teratogenicity
Barbiturates	Tonic-clonic seizures	Drowsiness, Unsteadiness	Rashes	Tolerance Habituation Withdrawal seizures Behavioural change	Confirmed in man and animals
Phenytoin	Tonic-clonic seizures	Unsteadiness Slurred speech Chorea	Rashes Lymphadenopathy Hepatitis	Gum swelling Acne Hirsutism Folate deficiency	Confirmed in man and animals
Carbamazepine	Partial epilepsy +/- 2y generalisation	Dizziness Diplopia Unsteadiness Nausea Vomiting	Rashes Low white cell count	? None definite	Confirmed in man and animals
Sodium valproate	Idiopathic generalised + partial epilepsy	Tremor Irritability Restlessness Occasional confusion	Gastric intolerance Hepatotoxicity (in children)	? Weight gain Alopecia	Confirmed in man and animals

Table 2 The new anti-epileptic drugs.

	Mode of action	Efficacy in seizure type (mode of use)	Adverse events		Teratogenicity
			Acute idiosyncratic	Chronic toxicity	
Eslicarbazepine	Na channel block	Partial (add-on)	Hyponatraemia	-	Unknown
Felbamate	Glycine antagonism	Partial / generalised (monotherapy / add-on)	Bone marrow suppression Hepatic failure	-	Unknown
Gabapentin	Uncertain ?GABAergic effect ?Ca channel block	Partial (add-on)	Behavioural problems (children)	-	None described as yet
Lacosamide	Na channel block	Partial (add-on)	-	-	Unknown
Lamotrigine	Na channel block	Partial / generalised (monotherapy/add-on)	Rash	-	None described as yet
Levetiracetam	Unknown	Partial / ?generalised (add-on)	-	-	None described as yet
Oxcarbazepine	Na channel block Ca channel block	Partial (add-on / monotherapy)	-	Hyponatraemia	Unknown
Rufinamide	Unknown	Add-on for refractory Lennox-Gastaut	-	-	Unknown
Tiagabine	GABA reuptake block	Partial (add-on)	Partial status	-	Animal models
Topiramate	GABAergic Na channel block Kainate receptor block	Partial / generalised (add-on / monotherapy)	-	Renal calculi Weight loss	Animal models
Vigabatrin	GABA-t inhibition	Partial (add-on)	Psychosis	Visual field defects	Animal models
Zonisamide	Na channel block	Partial / ?generalised (add-on / ?monotherapy)	-	Renal calculi	Animal models and isolated case reports in humans

Barbiturates

Although barbiturates have a wide range of effects on many neurobiological systems, their main anti-epileptic effect derives from their specific binding to the $GABA_A$ receptor which increases the frequency of chloride channel opening, and thereby increases membrane stability in the nervous system.

Phenobarbitone and primidone are the two barbiturates most commonly used in clinical practice. The Veterans' Administration study run by Mattson *et al* in the mid-eighties confirmed that barbiturates are not as well tolerated as their newer counterparts.

Phenobarbitone

Phenobarbitone is active against partial and generalised tonic-clonic seizures, as well as in prevention of febrile seizures and treatment of some cases of status epilepticus. Development of tolerance can also prove problematical, while the risk of withdrawal seizures mean that patients whose seizures are well controlled on phenobarbitone should not have their treatment altered unless there is good reason.

Phenobarbitone is an inexpensive anticonvulsant, and will therefore remain important in developing countries. In the developed world, where cost is less of a determining factor, it will remain less attractive than its better-tolerated successors.

Primidone

Primidone is a barbiturate pro-drug (converted in the liver to phenobarbitone), which is less effective and less well tolerated than carbamazepine, phenytoin or phenobarbitone. The most common side effects are drowsiness, gastro-intestinal intolerance and psychosis. Physical dependence and withdrawal seizures are also barriers to long-term use.

Benzodiazepines

Benzodiazepines exert their anticonvulsant effect on binding with a specific site on the $GABA_A$ receptor, which increases hyperpolarisation of affected neurones. Additionally, some effects on sodium channels have been described.

Benzodiazepines, such as diazepam and lorazepam, still have a place in the immediate, intravenous treatment of status epilepticus. Clobazam is less sedative than the older benzodiazepines and can be useful when given as adjunctive treatment. While intermittent treatment is more common with benzodiazepines, some studies have supported the long-term use of clonazepam and clorazepate.

Bromide salts

Bromide salts act by potentiating the action of GABA on the chloride channel. The high incidence of sedation and dermatological side effects have ensured that bromides are considered for use in only the most refractory of epilepsies.

Carbamazepine

Carbamazepine is a tricyclic compound which has been available since the 1960s. It remains a first-line AED for the treatment of localisation-related epilepsies. Carbamazepine has a wide range of neurochemical and neurophysiological actions: sodium channel blockade, which limits sustained repetitive firing, is probably the most important, but many other synaptic effects have been described. Until publication of the SANAD study, carbamazepine was considered to be the drug of choice for partial epilepsies, but the suggestion of a reduced incidence of side effects with lamotrigine has made this, in many people's opinion, a first choice instead. It has no documented efficacy against generalised absences or myoclonic seizures, and in fact the latter seizure type may on occasion be exacerbated by carbamazepine.

Although generally well tolerated, carbamazepine's pharmacokinetics may be disadvantageous, leading to marked inter- and intra-individual variation in response. Rashes and hyponatraemia may occur in some patients. The incidence and severity of the neurological side effects (nausea, headache, dizziness and diplopia) correlate with the levels of both carbamazepine and its active metabolite, carbamazepine-epoxide.

Carbamazepine's success as an anti-epileptic drug has been augmented by the development of the slow release preparation, which leads to an increased tolerability via a decrease in plasma level variability.

Eslicarbazepine

Eslicarbazepine is a modified form of carbamazepine. This drug has a different pharmacology, and the production of breakdown products differs from those produced with carbamazepine. This recently licensed medication is therefore of use in patients who have had good therapeutic efficacy from carbamazepine, but could not tolerate the adverse effects, many of which come from breakdown products, such as the epoxide derivatives of carbamazepine.

Ethosuximide and other succinimides

The succinimides were synthesised to be modifications of the hydantoin-barbiturate heterocyclic ring. Ethosuximide is the most commonly used succinimide, the other two (methsuximide and phensuximide) being little used today. Ethosuximide remains a useful compound in paediatric practice in the treatment of absence seizures but (unlike some other succinimides) it does not appear to be effective against other seizure types. Side effects of ethosuximide are either gastro-intestinal (nausea, vomiting, abdominal pain) or involve the central nervous system (lethargy, dizziness, ataxia).

Ethosuximide does not alter the metabolism of other drugs, but its own metabolism is affected by enzyme-inducing or inhibiting anti-epileptic drugs. The efficacy and safety of valproate has ensured that ethosuximide has become a second-line treatment for absence seizures.

Felbamate

Felbamate is structurally unrelated to other anticonvulsant compounds, and was approved for use in adults in the USA in 1992, with subsequent approval given for use in children with Lennox-Gastaut syndrome.

Add-on studies demonstrated felbamate's efficacy in intractable focal seizures, while two trials showed efficacy as monotherapy during withdrawal of conventional AEDs. Most side effects were attributed to the interaction of felbamate with concomitant AEDs. However, by 1995, after around 100,000 felbamate exposures, two very serious problems arose: aplastic anaemia had developed in 32 patients, and hepatic failure in 19 patients. Five of those with hepatotoxicity, and ten of those with bone marrow suppression have died.

Current use is generally restricted to those patients refractory to all other medications and in whom the risk-benefit relationship is favourable. Weekly or bi-weekly blood counts and liver function tests must be performed, although it is not clear whether early detection of either of these idiosyncratic reactions will prevent the most serious outcomes.

Gabapentin

Gabapentin was developed in an attempt to manufacture a direct GABA receptor agonist that could be administered orally. In fact, the full neurobiological effects of gabapentin have not yet been clearly defined, although it is likely that it binds to a subunit of the calcium channel protein. It has also been suggested that gabapentin could alter transport of other neurotransmitter amino acids *in vivo*.

Gabapentin is excreted unchanged by the kidneys and has no known drug interactions. Studies showed gabapentin to be effective at rather lower doses than are currently used. Compared to the upper end of the licensed doses in most countries, the studied doses of 900mg/day or 1200mg/day seem rather low. Despite this, these studies confirmed the drug's efficacy as add-on therapy against refractory partial epilepsy.

In clinical trials, gabapentin has been very well tolerated; adverse events are relatively rare and there are no reports of any life-threatening side effects of gabapentin use. Comparison with other monotherapies in the SANAD studies suggested that this drug has less efficacy as monotherapy than others, leading to less uptake in use. The most common side effects are somnolence, fatigue, dizziness and weight gain. Gabapentin is also widely used in the management of chronic pain syndromes.

Lacosamide

Lacosamide is a new anti-epileptic drug which has a specific action on neuronal sodium channels. Oral absorption is rapid and the elimination half-life is around 13 hours. There are no definite drug interactions. Efficacy has been shown as adjunctive treatment against partial epilepsy. The most common side effects are dizziness, headache, nausea and diplopia. These tend to occur during titration. Since being licensed, lacosamide has been a helpful drug in boosting control in patients refractory to other medications.

Lamotrigine

In the 1960s, some AED development programmes concentrated on antagonism of proconvulsive compounds such as folate. Lamotrigine is chemically unrelated to other AEDs, and was noted to be both a mild folate antagonist and anticonvulsant when used in some animal models. It is now known that these properties are not linked.

Lamotrigine inhibits neuronal burst firing in a manner similar to that of phenytoin and carbamazepine, but also helps block sustained repetitive firing as a result of sodium channel inactivation. This occurs when the channel is at the slow inactivated state, and this selectivity may account for the drug's tolerability.

Lamotrigine metabolism is largely hepatic, but lamotrigine does not induce or inhibit hepatic enzymes. There may be a pharmacodynamic interaction with carbamazepine which results in an increase in neurotoxicity when the drugs are combined. Lamotrigine's half-life is extended by concomitant valproate, while enzyme-inducing anticonvulsants such as carbamazepine and phenytoin have the opposite effect. There is a mutual interaction with synthetic oestrogens with each increasing breakdown of the other. Therefore, caution with epilepsy and contraceptive control has to be exercised (requiring larger doses of both drugs when used together).

The SANAD study compared lamotrigine monotherapy with other monotherapies in partial epilepsy. In that study, lamotrigine showed similar efficacy but improved tolerability compared with carbamazepine, topiramate and gabapentin. The drug is also licensed for use in Lennox-Gastaut syndrome and idiopathic generalised epilepsies. In the SANAD arm looking at generalised epilepsies, however, the efficacy was less than with valproate and topiramate. Despite this, the drug may have a role in newly diagnosed generalised epilepsies given that it does not have the same profile of teratogenesis and difficulties with prenatal exposure seen with valproate and topiramate.

Skin rash and mild central nervous system events, such as dizziness, ataxia, drowsiness, headache and diplopia occur with lamotrigine use.

Levetiracetam

Levetiracetam is chemically related to piracetam, a nootropic drug, but is not structurally similar to any existing AED. The mechanism of action of levetiracetam relies on binding to intracellular proteins.

Initial studies demonstrated efficacy in refractory partial seizures in man, while later studies have also shown efficacy in animal models of idiopathic generalised epilepsy. Such effects have led to its increasing use as monotherapy in both partial and generalised epilepsies. Levetiracetam's pharmacokinetics are linear, and no interactions have been described with other drugs. Long-term comparative studies of levetiracetam have still to be completed, but it would appear that the efficacy and excellent tolerability will make this drug a mainstay of anti-epileptic drug treatment in the 21st century.

Oxcarbazepine

Oxcarbazepine is a chemical analogue of carbamazepine with a radically different metabolic profile. The mechanism of action of oxcarbazepine is closely related to that of carbamazepine; its major effect is in preventing repetitive firing of neurones by blocking voltage-dependent Na^+ channels. There may be some differences in effects, and one trial demonstrated that oxcarbazepine could prove beneficial on being added into a regime containing carbamazepine without provoking toxicity. Oxcarbazepine does not result in auto-induction or hepatic enzyme induction, and there is no interaction with the oral contraceptive pill. The converse does not apply, however, as enzyme induction by other AEDs decreases hydroxy-carbamazepine concentrations.

A number of trials support the idea that the two compounds have similar efficacy against partial epilepsy, but like carbamazepine, it is ineffective against idiopathic generalised epilepsies. The SANAD study used oxcarbazepine latterly in its comparative arm in partial epilepsy with demonstration of comparable efficacy and tolerability.

Side effects are similar to those produced by carbamazepine; dizziness, drowsiness, headache, nausea, vomiting and diplopia are the most prominent symptoms. Studies have reported these to be less frequent and less severe than with carbamazepine. In addition, oxcarbazepine produces fewer rashes and perhaps fewer idiosyncratic reactions. Hyponatraemia is more common with oxcarbazepine than with carbamazepine, but is usually mild and asymptomatic.

Phenytoin

Phenytoin has been used worldwide since its introduction in 1938. Laboratory studies have demonstrated phenytoin's effect on many facets of neuronal physiology and biochemistry. It is unlikely that any one single action is the source of its anticonvulsant activity, and it is more probable that this depends on a combination of its many effects.

Phenytoin has marked activity against partial seizures with or without secondary generalisation. In some developed countries, particularly the USA, it remains a drug of choice for idiopathic generalised epilepsies. Intravenous phenytoin is still considered the treatment of choice for status epilepticus not fully responsive to benzodiazepines.

The pharmacokinetics exhibited by phenytoin ensure that it demands careful monitoring during dose titration, particularly when used as part of AED polypharmacy. In clinical practice this need for monitoring is a distinct disadvantage.

Chronic phenytoin use can cause hirsutism, gum hyperplasia and facial coarsening. Such cosmetic effects can make the drug less useful in young women. CNS features of phenytoin toxicity include cognitive decline and cerebellar ataxia. Interference with metabolism of folate or vitamin D can result in a mild macrocytic anaemia or osteomalacia, respectively. There is a recognised risk of fetal abnormality with phenytoin treatment, although the risks to the fetus of uncontrolled epilepsy would justify its use in some pregnancies.

Pregabalin

Pregabalin was a chemical modification of gabapentin, and has been shown to have higher potency at the same binding site on the α2-delta subunit of the calcium channel. This chemical modification is also associated with additional mechanisms of action compared to gabapentin. In addition to its role as an anti-epileptic drug, pregabalin has been given a licence for use as an anti-anxiety medication. Patients on treatment with pregabalin are said to have improved sleep hygiene and improved depression scores. Since anxiety and depression are common comorbidities of epilepsy, such side benefits may be important in helping to choose pregabalin over other adjunctive therapies, especially in patients with primary cerebral neoplasms, where there may be a predisposition to anxiety.

Side effects of pregablin include weight gain and fluid retention. No significant drug interactions have been described.

Progabide

Progabide is a direct GABA receptor agonist which underwent clinical evaluation in the 1980s. Conflicting results from these studies, and a continuing risk of hepatotoxicity, have combined to stop the drug being used outwith France.

Retigabine

Retigabine is a new drug which has been shown to have a different action on sodium channels from other anti-epileptic drugs. Initial studies would suggest that some patients resistant to the older AEDs will receive significant benefit from retigabine. Dizziness and drowsiness are recognised side effects of this medication.

Rufinamide

Rufinamide has been granted a licence for use as an adjunctive treatment in patients with Lennox-Gastaut syndrome. Trials have shown it to be useful in preventing generalised or drop attacks. It retains a limited indication.

Sulthiame

Sulthiame is chemically related to acetazolamide, but has been shown to have a greater inhibitory effect on the neuronal isoenzyme of carbonic anhydrase. It was first used in Europe and Australia as adjunctive treatment of partial and generalised seizures with some success. Monotherapy trials showed the compound to be less well tolerated than the established AEDs. Sulthiame cannot be considered to be a first choice of AED.

Tiagabine

Tiagabine inhibits GABA reuptake into neurones and glial cells, so enhancing the synaptic levels and effects of GABA. The large addition to the nipecotic acid molecule helps the compound to cross the blood-brain barrier following oral administration.

Patients on a regime containing enzyme-inducing drugs metabolise tiagabine at a faster rate. Co-administration of tiagabine does not have an effect on the pharmacokinetics of concomitant AEDs. Clinical studies have confirmed the efficacy of this compound against partial seizures with or without secondary generalisation.

Tolerability seemed to compare favourably with the established AEDs. Most adverse events are mild, but some reports have suggested an increase in the incidence of complex partial status at higher doses, but a particular association has not been confirmed statistically.

Topiramate

Topiramate is chemically unrelated to other AEDs, deriving as it does from D-fructose. It is likely that, like established AEDs, the anticonvulsant activity depends on a combination of effects on sodium channels, carbonic anhydrase, calcium channels and GABA receptors.

Topiramate pharmacokinetics are linear, the plasma level increasing in proportion to the dose. Established enzyme-inducing AEDs increase the clearance of topiramate. The clearance of both digoxin and oestrogen are increased by topiramate.

Trials of efficacy in partial and generalised epilepsies have shown the benefits of topiramate at doses up to 1000mg/day. The drug has also been used as monotherapy, resulting in licence extensions in recent years. The SANAD studies confirmed the drug's usefulness in both localisation-related and generalised epilepsies.

The most commonly described adverse events include ataxia, dizziness, poor concentration, asthenia, paraesthesiae and weight loss. Nephrolithiasis occurs more commonly during treatment with topiramate, and the drug is best avoided in those with a family history of renal calculi.

No specific relationship with human teratogenicity has been determined, and the drug should only be used during pregnancy where it is felt that the benefit is greater than any potential risks.

Valproic acid

The exact mechanism by which sodium valproate exerts its anticonvulsant effect is unknown, but it has several actions which may contribute, including effects on the GABAergic system and on sodium channels.

Valproate's efficacy has been confirmed against generalised and partial epilepsies. Myoclonic epilepsy and absence attacks are effectively treated by valproate. Valproate does not induce hepatic enzymes, and since neither efficacy nor toxicity of valproate can be correlated with plasma levels, serum level monitoring is not necessary with valproate monotherapy. Drug interactions are less troublesome than with enzyme-inducing AEDs, although it does possess some enzyme-inhibiting properties. This is of clinical significance when the drug is added to existing anticonvulsant treatment regimes, particularly those containing lamotrigine.

Adverse effects include tremor, hair loss and weight gain. Dose reduction may partially solve these, but withdrawal of the drug may be necessary. There is a recognised risk of teratogenicity with valproate use, although the subsequent risk to childhood cognition (part of the so-called fetal valproate syndrome) is an evolving story which may further reduce use of this drug in women of child-bearing age. Rare, though more serious, are episodes of hepatitis, hepatic failure, pancreatitis, thrombocytopenia and coma which have been associated. Serious adverse effects are more common in children, but their rarity has ensured that valproate is still considered to be safe. Use of the compound in countries such as the USA is still limited as a result of concerns regarding these adverse effects.

Vigabatrin

Vigabatrin is structurally very similar to GABA, and was the first 'designer' AED, i.e. a drug specifically designed to enhance a single biochemical action. Initial promise was hampered by psychiatric adverse effects when the starting dose was high and titration rapid. Description of asymptomatic visual field defects in 1998 led to further restrictions in use, and vigabatrin is now rarely used without prior assessment of visual fields and regular monitoring.

Vigabatrin binds to the enzyme responsible for GABA breakdown, an irreversible covalent bond which inactivates GABA-transaminase. This mechanism of action inspired the descriptive term 'suicide inhibitor' of GABA-T. Resultant increases in GABA levels lead to an augmentation of neuronal inhibition.

Vigabatrin is rapidly absorbed after oral administration and the majority of each dose is excreted unchanged in the urine. The plasma half-life is around 8 hours, but the mode of action ensures that the pharmacological effect of vigabatrin is much longer than its pharmacokinetic half-life.

As would be expected, no clinically important interactions with other anticonvulsants have been described. Many studies have confirmed the efficacy of vigabatrin as add-on therapy for refractory epilepsy in adults. Good monotherapy evidence has never been established, and the drug is indicated in adults only for partial epilepsies as adjunctive therapy. In children, vigabatrin has been shown to be superior to steroids in the treatment of infantile spasms (West syndrome).

The most common side effects are those of dizziness, headache, diplopia, ataxia and vertigo. Psychiatric side effects such as anxiety, depression and aggression are well recognised; the precipitation of psychosis at a high dose or following sudden withdrawal of the drug should lead to cautious use of vigabatrin in those with a history of psychiatric illness.

Zonisamide

Zonisamide's actions in blocking sodium and calcium channels may help explain its effects in a number of animal models of epilepsy. The drug also has some inhibitory effect on carbonic anhydrase.

Studies have shown benefit in both localisation-related and idiopathic generalised epilepsies. The drug undergoes hepatic metabolism, and enzyme-inducing AEDs reduce plasma concentrations when used concurrently. Drowsiness and ataxia are the most common side effects, occurring with both monotherapy and polypharmacy. Renal calculus formation is more prominent in European and US-based studies, than in Japanese populations.

Teratogenic effects were noted in various species at higher doses, but there are only isolated case reports of human teratogenicity when zonisamide is part of a regime of AED polypharmacy. The drug is recommended for use during pregnancy only if the therapeutic benefit outweighs the potential risks.

Possible future treatments

There are a number of new anti-epileptic drugs under development (see Chapter 9). While increasing the numbers of available AEDs may make the non-specialist's heart sink, it should make some of us more hopeful that we can come clearer to our goal of finding a specific treatment for specific epilepsies. Merely increasing drug numbers will not be enough; we need to find ways of evaluating and predicting responses of individual patients to specific drugs.

Conclusions

There is a huge expansion in the number of drugs available for epilepsy. Most people respond well to treatment, but the newer drugs give us a better chance of long-term control with fewer side effects.

Key Summary

◆ Don't be bewildered by the range of AEDs on offer.

◆ Few are used routinely.

◆ The choice of drug depends on epilepsy type.

◆ Newer drugs are arriving all the time.

◆ Each progress in epilepsy means more hope for patients.

References

1. Mattson RH, Cramer RH, Collins JF, *et al*. Comparison of carbamazepine, phenobarbital, phenytoin, and primidone in partial and secondarily generalized tonic-clonic seizures. *New England Journal of Medicine* 1985; 313: 145-51.

2. Marson AG, Al-Kharusi AM, Alwaidh M, Appleton R, Baker GA, Chadwick DW, Cramp C, Cockerell OC, Cooper P, Doughty J, Eaton B, Gamble C, Goulding RP, Howell SJL, Hughes A, Jackson M, Jacoby A, Kellett M, Lawson GR, Leach JP, Nicolaides P, Roberts R, Shackley P, Shen J, Smith DF, Smith PEM, Tudur-Smith C, Vanoli A, Williamson PR. The SANAD study of effectiveness of valproate, lamotrigine, or topiramate for generalised and unclassifiable epilepsy: an unblinded randomised controlled trial. *Lancet* 2007; 369: 1016-26.

3. Marson AG, Al-Kharusi AM, Alwaidh M, Appleton R, Baker GA, Chadwick DW, Cramp C, Cockerell OC, Cooper P, Doughty J, Eaton B, Gamble C, Goulding RP, Howell SJL, Hughes A, Jackson M, Jacoby A, Kellett M, Lawson GR, Leach JP, Nicolaides P,

Roberts R, Shackley P, Shen J, Smith DF, Smith PEM, Tudur-Smith C, Vanoli A, Williamson PR. The SANAD study of effectiveness of carbamazepine, gabapentin, lamotrigine, oxcarbazepine, or topiramate for treatment of partial epilepsy: an unblinded randomised controlled trial. *Lancet* 2007; 369: 1000-15.

4.   Levy RH, Mattson RH, Meldrum B, Perrucca E. *Antiepileptic Drugs*, 5th ed. Philadelphia, USA: Lippincott, Williams and Wilkins, 2002.

5.   Patsalos PN, Perucca E. Clinically important drug interactions in epilepsy: general features and interactions between antiepileptic drugs. *Lancet Neurology* 2003; 2: 347-56.

6.   Patsalos PN, Perucca E. Clinically important drug interactions in epilepsy: general features and interactions between antiepileptic drugs and other drugs. *Lancet Neurology* 2003; 2: 473-81.

Chapter 9
Future developments in the treatment of epilepsy

The list of anti-epileptic drugs continues to expand. While the non-specialist may view this with some dismay, patients and their families may feel a sense of hope. Whether any of these new compounds will in themselves change the remission risk is of course uncertain. It could be argued that instead of a relentless search for new compounds, we should learn to better use the ones already available.

Epilepsy is a condition which results from a host of predisposing and preventative factors. While some genes will alter the function of individual channels and make seizure activity more likely, there will also be some genes which have, by virtue of their effects on ion channels and neurotransmitters, anticonvulsant properties. The complexity of this disorder and the multiplicity of causes will explain the differing phenotypes in families with apparent 'single gene' epilepsies, and would also explain the differing response to drugs among apparently similar clinical syndromes.

Current clinical practice means that when a diagnosis has been made, treatment is chosen on an empirical basis. How can things improve for patients? How can we increase the chances of an early and complete response to AEDs?

Better drugs

There are a number of compounds undergoing investigation for use as anti-epileptic drugs. The most promising continue to be described in the biennial reports from the conference on emerging AEDs, the so-called Eilat conferences which have been taking place since the 1990s. If there is a theme from these new drugs, it is in recognition that the drugs have predictable pharmacokinetics, have few interactions, and possibly more excitingly, are not reliant on the same modes of action as the established drugs. The drugs most likely to obtain approval for use in clinics are listed below.

Licensed in some countries / states

Lacosamide

Lacosamide is a new anti-epileptic drug which has a specific action on neuronal sodium channels. Oral absorption is rapid and the elimination half-life is around 13 hours. There are no definite drug interactions. Efficacy has been shown as adjunctive treatment against partial epilepsy. The most common side effects are dizziness, headache, nausea and diplopia. These tend to occur during titration. Since being licensed, lacosamide has been a helpful drug in boosting control in patients refractory to other medications.

Eslicarbazepine

Eslicarbazepine is a modified tricyclic which has a different metabolic pathway from its forebear, carbamazepine. This avoids formation of epoxide derivatives of carbamazine, and reduces the incidence of side effects. The mode of action of eslicarbazepine is probably similar to that of carbamazepine. In humans, eslicarbazepine is rapidly absorbed, with linear and proportional metabolism unaffected by other AEDs.

Phase III studies have shown efficacy in refractory partial epilepsy. Treatment-related side effects were similar in nature to those with carbamazepine. Hyponatraemia remains a potential concern.

Potential new drugs awaiting approval

Brivaracetam

Brivaracetam, like its forebear levetiracetam, has an affinity for synaptic vesicle protein 2A (SV2A) albeit at a ten-times higher potency - this may affect exocytosis and neurotransmitter release. Brivaracetam also has additional effects on sodium channel action which may confer additional anticonvulsant action. *In vitro* and *in vivo* studies have confirmed the actions of brivaracetam in a wide range of seizure models.

Clinical studies in humans have confirmed complete and rapid absorption in humans, with hepatic metabolism and low protein binding. There is no tendency towards enzyme induction or inhibition. There appears to be no interaction with any other AEDs.

Efficacy has been studied in Phase II studies and full data from Phase II studies are awaited to demonstrate usefulness of this drug in patients with refractory partial epilepsy. Future work will be needed to confirm or refute an effect on generalised epilepsies as noted with levetiracetam. No serious adverse effects have been demonstrated at this early stage.

Carisbamate

Carisbamate is a novel anti-epileptic drug which has no chemical similarity with any other existing AEDs. Preclinical studies would suggest that the drug has action against both partial and generalised epilepsies, although the exact mode of action remains elusive. Human pharmacological studies show the drug to be rapidly and completely absorbed, with hepatic metabolism almost complete, and a minimal (probably clinically unimportant) tendency to effect change in metabolism of other AEDs. Enzyme-inducing AEDs will reduce exposure to activity of carisbamate. Hepatic impairment will give higher serum levels than in those with normal liver function.

Large Phase III studies are expected to explore the activity against refractory partial epilepsies. Further studies are expected in children and in patients with neuropathic pain.

Deoxyglucose

One of the fascinating developments in AEDs is in the assessment of this chemical analogue of glucose. The antiseizure effects of this compound were discovered during studies of neuronal activity during the ketogenic diet. It has been noted that carbohydrate ingestion reduced the anti-epileptic effect of the diet, and the tracer labelled deoxyglucose was being used to assess metabolism of monosaccharides. Preclinical studies have suggested a usefulness of 2-deoxyglucose (2-DG) in acute and chronic settings. Studies have failed to show an action on a single process or system, but there is an inhibition of glycolysis after administration of 2DG which may inhibit seizure onset and propagation.

Unsurprising, given the chemical similarity to glucose, the absorption and hepatic metabolism of 2-DG are consistent and unremarkable. Neurones with the highest metabolic rate (i.e. those with most seizure activity) are most avid in the uptake of glucose (and therefore 2-DG). Unlike glucose, 2-DG cannot undergo further metabolism once phosphatisation has occurred, meaning that the drug becomes 'trapped' once inside the neurones, leading to altered glucose metabolism and reduced metabolic activity. Early preclinical studies have not shown widespread long-term effects of acute usage of 2-DG. Future studies are planned to assess the effects of 2-DG on refractory epilepsy in humans.

Ganaxolone

Ganaxolone is an analogue of the neurosteroid allopregnalone. While having no demonstrable steroid activity, this drug modifies GABA receptor response, leaving protection against a wide range of seizure models in animals. There is also the possibility of having an effect on long-term epiletogenesis. In humans, ganaxolone is rapidly absorbed especially in the presence of ingested food, with a half-life of around 10 hours. Preliminary data would suggest there are no significant drug interactions and efficacy has been shown in small short-term studies in both adults and children. Side effects have so far been mild and short-lived, and further Phase III studies are awaited.

Huperzine

Huperzine is the active ingredient in Chinese folk medicine used against a number of diverse illnesses. There has been limited activity shown in animal models, but planned studies are anticipated in humans with refractory epilepsy of partial origin.

JZP-4

JZP-4 is a derivative of pyrazine diamine which has effects in blocking sodium and calcium channels. Animal studies have suggested that the drug may be useful in refractory partial epilepsy. Further studies in patients with tremor and neuropathic pain are planned. Most of the drug is excreted unchanged, and there has been no effect shown on metabolism of other AEDs. Small studies in humans have shown effects in reducing generalised discharges.

NAX-5055

NAX-5055 is an analogue of galanin, an endogenous neuropeptide, which has been shown to have an effect on induced seizures. NAX-5055 has been shown to have anti-epileptic effects in a wide range of seizure models when applied directly to the brain, in a unique pattern compared to other AEDs. Further studies in humans are required.

Propylisopropyl acetamide (PID)

This derivative of valproic acid was discovered during a search for potential AEDs. The promise in this drug lies in its lack of demonstrable teratogenesis. If the drug could retain the efficacy without the adverse effects of valproate, then there could be significant benefit in its use. Future studies are required to prove usefulness in epilepsy.

Retigabine

Retigabine is a compound which has undergone recent study in patients with refractory epilepsy. It has a unique site of action for an AED, increasing current in M-current in KCNQ (Kv7) potassium channels. Other actions were demonstrated on calcium channels and responsiveness of GABA receptors, but the relative contributions of these is uncertain.

Absorption in humans is rapid and complete. Preclinical studies have shown activity in models of partial and generalised epilepsy with linear hepatic metabolism. There is no effect on or by AEDs.

Phase III studies of a range of doses took place over a 12-week treatment phase, with halving of seizure frequency in 19-30%, more than in placebo-exposed patients, and seizure count reducing by a median of 18-30%, more than with placebo.

Dizziness, drowsiness and fatigue result from use of this drug, but no serious adverse effects have so far emerged.

T2000 - 1,3-dimethoxymethyl-5,5-diphenylbarbituric acid
There are two barbiturate derivatives which may undergo further studies. These diphenyl barbiturates are less sedative than other barbiturates.

Tonabersat
This is a chemical analogue of carabersat. It has a binding site across the frontal regions and hippocampus, with a 2-3 times greater affinity than carabersat. The effect is thought to be on gap junction sites, which have been unaffected in studies of all other AEDs. Conversely, tonabersat has not been shown to have any effect on traditional models of anticonvulsant effect - its effect is one that has been untapped in reducing seizures with traditional AEDs. Tonabersat is rapidly absorbed after ingestion in humans, and there is no evidence of hepatic enzyme induction. Although no interaction studies have been performed with other AEDs, there is no significant interaction with synthetic oestrogens or acute migraine treatments. Animal studies have shown some effect on several different models, suggesting effectiveness in partial epilepsy. Human studies have centred mostly on migraine, but this compound holds some promise as an AED.

Valrocemide
Valrocemide was initially developed as a valproate-linked GABA analogue. Animal studies have shown more potent activity than with

valproate. Pharmacokinetics are linear, with good absorption, and excretion of the compound is largely unchanged in the urine. Enzyme inducers increase glycination of valrocemide, perhaps enhancing effectiveness, and there is an absence of effect of valrocemide on the pharmacokinetics of other AEDs. Detailed Phase III studies are required to prove a significant effect of valrocemide on refractory epilepsy.

YKP3089

This novel compound has activity against a range of animal seizure models. Phase I and II studies have shown the compound to be well-tolerated, but more studies are required to prove efficacy in man.

Better use of existing drugs

Pharmacogenomics - improving drug selection

Since it is unlikely that we have the dose wrong, any improvement in their use will result from better selection of drugs in individual patients, with the knowledge to predict who will have less tendency to side effects from each drug, and which drug will best control the seizures. Such an aim has already led to the identification of a sodium channel gene allele that predicts an idiosyncratic reaction to carbamazepine. In time, genetic information may allow prediction of more subtle and less dramatic side effects.

In a similar vein, it can only be hoped that full genetic analysis would allow prediction of anti-epileptic response.

Improved delivery

Improving efficacy may mean helping to deliver drugs more closely to the time and place when seizure activity is most likely. Better temporal placement would involve automatic administration when seizure activity becomes apparent on an EEG, and there are systems which are being developed to detect and prevent seizures, which would trigger a bolus of anti-epileptic drug.

Additionally, some systems are in use which would allow for direct administration to the set of epileptic activity (e.g. intraventricular administration via an intracranial catheter).

Better combination

Among the main advantages of the newer AEDs is that they tend to have fairly straightforward pharmacokinetics; they have a far less tendency to cause induction of hepatic enzymes and mutual interactions are rare. Their variable modes of action could theoretically lead to an ability to combine drugs with different modes of action producing a synergy of anti-epileptic effect. Unfortunately, we are still no closer to establishing which is the most potent combination. An increasing number of drugs, of course, leads to an exponential increase in the number of possible combinations, making it more difficult for any particular combination to stand out. Large studies would be needed to prove superiority with any certainty, and it is unlikely that there is the will or the finance available to support such studies.

Other devices and surgery

The effects of intracranial and perineurological systems have been postulated for some time. The most common has been the vagal nerve stimulator. Despite its use as a licensed medical device for over 10 years, there remains a need for further work to explain, or expand upon the use, of such devices. While there are anecdotal studies suggesting efficacy, more information is still necessary to help justify and predict the usefulness of this device. Stimulation of other neurological centres may be found to have efficacy in future.

If there are to be advances in surgery in the coming years, they will require improvement of two processes: the elucidation of the epileptogenic zone where there is no lesion on imaging, and the ability to clearly separate the site of planned surgery from centres of functional importance. Improved use of EEG, utilising depth electrodes and recognition of particular discharges will help with the former, but the latter will need functional imaging techniques to continue to reassure neurosurgeons that intervention will not cause significant deficits in speech or memory.

Conclusions

For many years, patients with epilepsy and their clinicians have had to accept that there is a continued inability to control seizures in a significant minority. In the last 20 years, with the introduction of a dozen or so drugs, this incidence of refractory epilepsy has been static. Hopefully things may be changing, and with better results from drugs, and better use of surgery, we may at last make inroads into those patients with continued epilepsy.

Key Summary

◆ Given the significant minority of patients with epilepsy who remain resistant to treatment, we need to improve treatment.

◆ Drug effectiveness may be improved by targeting times and sites of greatest need or better combining the drugs to maximise efficacy and minimise side effects.

◆ New drugs may help reduce seizures by using previously untapped mechanisms of action.

◆ There remains significant room for technology in improving safety and availability of surgery.

References

1. Bialera M, *et al.* Progress report on new antiepileptic drugs: a summary of the Ninth Eilat Conference (EILAT IX). *Epilepsy Research* 2009; 83: 1-43.

Chapter 10
When things go well - monotherapy and withdrawal

Choosing monotherapy with anti-epileptic drugs

It is usual for patients with newly diagnosed epilepsy to do well on treatment. The first AED trial will render 47% seizure-free. Of those remaining, around a third (around 15% of the total) will become seizure-free with the addition of a second AED, and 9% with a third. While studies have struggled to show that the response rate will be significantly higher with the newer drugs, there is a consistent trend in showing that newer drugs are better tolerated than their older counterparts. This is a significant boon to patients who have to take daily medications for a paroxysmal disorder, and it is likely that this improved tolerability will also prove a boon in improving adherence. With no clear winner in terms of response rates, initial monotherapy choice depends on several factors. It is important that drug choice is made after full discussion with the patient; such discussion is likely to focus on the likely prognosis, potential benefits and drawbacks of each treatment. Provision of this information will help the patient stick with the treatment and withstand temporary side effects. Such motivation is the first step in improving long-term patient compliance.

What drug to choose?

There is a lack of direct comparative data. The largest study in epilepsy care has been the SANAD (Standard and New Anti-epileptic Drugs) study, which was conceived as a pragmatic, prospective randomised study comparing efficacy and tolerability of standard treatment and new AEDs. This has informed choice of monotherapy in newly diagnosed epilepsy.

Partial epilepsy

Arm A of the SANAD study looked at patients with partial onset epilepsy, comparing the outcome in over a thousand patients treated with carbamazepine, lamotrigine, gabapentin, topiramate and oxcarbazepine. In the primary outcome measure of time to treatment failure, lamotrigine was less likely to fail for any reason compared to carbamazepine, topiramate and gabapentin. Gabapentin was significantly more likely to fail because of lack of efficacy than any of the other drugs, while withdrawal due to intolerable adverse effects was most frequently observed with carbamazepine and topiramate. Meta-analysis of five monotherapy RCTs showed lamotrigine to be significantly less likely to be withdrawn than carbamazepine.

Generalised epilepsy

Arm B of the SANAD study compared valproate (the 'gold standard' treatment for idiopathic generalised epilepsy) with lamotrigine and topiramate in the treatment of generalised and unclassified epilepsy. Of the three, valproate was significantly superior to lamotrigine and topiramate for the primary endpoints of time to treatment failure and time to 12-month seizure freedom. Lamotrigine was least efficacious, and topiramate was worst tolerated.

In keeping with SANAD, many clinicians (in the UK at least) would use lamotrigine or carbamazepine for partial epilepsies and valproate where the epilepsy is idiopathic generalised or unclassified, especially in males. The provision of information about the condition is as important as inclusion in the process of choosing medication; both processes will help empower the patient and leave them more able to face the hurdles presented by this condition. Where medical resources are scarce, the help presented by specialist nurses may be vital. The increasing demand for informed support will prove difficult to ignore in the coming years.

Furthermore, five new AEDs (levetiracetam, pregabalin, lacosamide, eslicarbazepine and zonisamide) were licensed in the UK since the initiation of the SANAD study, and the place of these drugs in newly diagnosed epilepsy is not addressed in SANAD. Of these new drugs, only levetiracetam has gained widespread usage as monotherapy in newly diagnosed epilepsy, but further studies are required to put the efficacy of these new drugs in context.

Response to initial monotherapy in newly diagnosed epilepsy

The diagnosis of epilepsy can have a devastating impact on patients. The ramifications are not only related to health, but also to social and economic implications. For the majority, the onset of epilepsy leads to several lifestyle restrictions, while the unpredictable and uncontrollable nature of seizures can engender a potentially debilitating sense of 'loss of control'. Seizure sequelae such as incontinence can also be a source of embarrassment, further worsening restricted social activity and isolation.

Loss of driving privileges is probably the most frequent cause for concern for adult patients and can have a significant impact on quality of life for patients in the developed world. Furthermore, loss of some employment types may have significant financial effects.

Studies examining response to AED treatment in newly diagnosed epilepsy generally paint an encouraging picture. Long-term remission is the norm in epilepsy, with the response to first drug proving prognostically useful. For patients failing initial monotherapy due to adverse effects, the subsequent chance of remission was similar to that in a drug naïve population, whereas failure due to lack of efficacy signified a worse outcome. Incomplete response to two drugs signalled a 90% chance, respectively, of remaining uncontrolled.

A family history of epilepsy, prior febrile seizures, traumatic brain injury, intermittent recreational drug use and psychiatric comorbidity were associated with a poorer response. Studies have suggested that a large number of seizures before starting treatment was a poor prognostic indicator, raising the question of whether repeated seizures themselves can lead to refractory epilepsy.

Overall, the trial data is not strong enough to support the immediate choice of any single AED for all new patients with epilepsy. Given the relatively high response rates for newly diagnosed epilepsy, it will take massive trials to be definite about the statistical differences required to make such a statement. Since there is no unanimous winner, a number of factors have to be taken into consideration when prescribing, for example, seizure classification, concomitant medication, side effects, fertility and side benefits.

Seizure classification
As described above, the choice of drug will be heavily influenced by the epilepsy classification. All drugs will have effect in partial epilepsy, while treatment of generalised epilepsy is restricted to lamotrigine, levetiracetam, topiramate, and valproate.

Concomitant medication
Where the patient is already on medication, the choice of an enzyme-inducing AED may reduce their effectiveness. Such interactions could prove life-threatening (e.g. with warfarin) or life-changing (e.g. with oestrogen-containing contraceptives).

Side effects
Where other medical conditions are present, the side effect profile of some AEDs may prove problematical (e.g. valproate-induced weight gain in patients with diabetes or asthma).

Fertility
Where the patient may be considering pregnancy in the future, some AEDs may frustrate this desire by reducing fertility (e.g. valproate) or may be potentially hazardous to the fetus. While much attention has rightly been placed on the risks of teratogenesis, it has become increasingly

apparent that some drugs may have selective effects on childhood development – a story that will undoubtedly progress in time.

Side benefits

Where comorbidities are present, whether these are related to the seizure disorder (such as anxiety, depression) or unrelated (such as obesity, neuropathic pain, or migraine), then some AEDs can prove helpful in their treatment.

When to stop treatment

It seems that paediatric neurologists are much more likely to stop treatment: this may tell us something (I'm not sure what) about epilepsy in children and its likelihood of remission.

Patients who have been seizure-free may have approached their doctor to ask about treatment cessation, often having been told that "If it ain't broke, don't fix it". While this may be true, it is much more useful if the decision is taken in the light of available evidence.

The best source of evidence comes from the MRC Drug Withdrawal Study and has been usefully summarised in tables included in the SIGN Guidelines (SIGN guideline number 70, pages 14-16). Factors shown to influence the risk of recurrence include the:

- duration of remission;
- pre-treatment EEG;
- number of drugs needed to control seizures;
- occurrence of any seizures after AED therapy was commenced;
- type of seizures experienced.

The use of these tables will give the patient an idea of relative recurrence risks, but such figures will not in themselves give absolutely firm pointers towards the best course of action. The patient will have a view on the desirability of drug withdrawal, a view very much determined by the patient's reaction to having a daily drug schedule, the presence of drug-related side effects, the social effects of any seizure recurrence (childcare, driving, employment), and the psychological and physical reaction to seizure recurrence (previous anxious depressive reaction, previous seizure-related trauma).

Patients will usually at some level have considered these, but may benefit from having them overtly discussed. The doctor's role in treatment cessation is to inform the patient about the risk of seizure recurrence on and off treatment. The decision to stop should be taken largely by the patient. Ultimately, such discussion will make a decision clear. If in doubt, the best policy is to keep the drug regime unchanged, leaving any decision about treatment cessation to be revisited at a future clinic appointment.

Conclusions

In summary, the choice of monotherapy depends mostly on a good classification of epilepsy. Other considerations (e.g. fertility) will play a part in the decision. Epilepsy treatment need not be for life, but withdrawal of drugs should be the patient's choice, a choice made once they have been made aware of the risks and benefits of drug withdrawal.

Key Summary

◆ Doing well is the most common outcome.

◆ Most will do well with a single AED.

◆ When things have gone well for a few years, patients may wish to come off treatment.

◆ They need good information to do this.

References

1. Marson AG, Al-Kharusi AM, Alwaidh M, Appleton R, Baker GA, Chadwick DW, Cramp C, Cockerell OC, Cooper P, Doughty J, Eaton B, Gamble C, Goulding RP, Howell SJL, Hughes A, Jackson M, Jacoby A, Kellett M, Lawson GR, Leach JP, Nicolaides P, Roberts R, Shackley P, Shen J, Smith DF, Smith PEM, Tudur-Smith C, Vanoli A, Williamson PR. The SANAD study of effectiveness of valproate, lamotrigine, or topiramate for generalised and unclassifiable epilepsy: an unblinded randomised controlled trial. *Lancet* 2007; 369: 1016-26.
2. Marson AG, Al-Kharusi AM, Alwaidh M, Appleton R, Baker GA, Chadwick DW, Cramp C, Cockerell OC, Cooper P, Doughty J, Eaton B, Gamble C, Goulding RP, Howell SJL, Hughes A, Jackson M, Jacoby A, Kellett M, Lawson GR, Leach JP, Nicolaides P, Roberts R, Shackley P, Shen J, Smith DF, Smith PEM, Tudur-Smith C, Vanoli A, Williamson PR. The SANAD study of effectiveness of carbamazepine, gabapentin, lamotrigine, oxcarbazepine, or topiramate for treatment of partial epilepsy: an unblinded randomised controlled trial. *Lancet* 2007; 369: 1000-15.
3. Kwan P, Brodie MJ. Early identification of refractory epilepsy. *N Engl J Med* 2000; 342: 314-9.
4. Chadwick D, for the Medical Research Council Antiepileptic Drug Withdrawal Study Group. Randomised study of antiepileptic drug withdrawal in patients in remission. *Lancet* 1991; 337: 1175-80.
5. SIGN 70 - Guidelines on diagnosis and treatment of epilepsy (www.sign.ac.uk).

Chapter 11
When things are not going well - polypharmacy, surgery and status epilepticus

Polypharmacy with AEDs - when good epilepsy goes bad

Most patients with epilepsy respond to the first or second AED. Studies confirm that remission rates are higher in idiopathic generalised epilepsy (IGE) than in those with partial epilepsy. Patients with an immediate good drug response are likely to remain seizure-free. Since such patients will be discharged after a few years, epilepsy clinics accumulate those patients who do not respond to medication, giving many neurologists an unrepresentative view of epilepsy outcome.

Early identification of drug-resistant patients is important, since this will allow the rapid use of drug combinations, targeting of investigations, work-up for epilepsy surgery, and the provision of specific information.

If seizures are not being completely controlled by medication, there are a series of questions that should be asked to identify if the epilepsy is genuinely refractory (Table 1). As listed below, these questions may highlight any quick solutions to the continuing episodes.

Correct diagnosis

Increasing specialist services have led to a decrease in the misdiagnosis rates. Misdiagnosis of epilepsy of around 20-25% has been demonstrated in both the hospital and the community. It should not be taken for granted that all 'events' are seizures, and a full description should

Table 1 Questions to ask when things are not going well.

- Correct diagnosis?

- Correct classification?

- Correct drug?

- Covert lesion?

- Compliance?

- Comorbidity?

- Confounding factors?

- Consistent with the truth?

be obtained for each type of event to ensure that the continuing episodes are potentially controlled by anti-epileptic drug treatment.

Correct classification

Even where the diagnosis of epilepsy is secure, the classification may be wrong, or may not have been considered. Patients with an IGE will be less likely to respond to sodium channel blockers such as carbamazepine or phenytoin and may in fact find their epilepsy exacerbated. Use of broad-spectrum AEDs such as lamotrigine or valproate will be necessary. Classification of epilepsy will often not be apparent on presentation, and may need to be reconsidered in the light of an EEG (if under 35 at onset), imaging, and any other emergent seizure types.

Covert lesion

Most patients will undergo cerebral imaging early, but where epilepsy is proving refractory, consideration and exclusion (with MRI) of a covert lesion is vital. This is particularly so where seizures are either unclassified or have a clinical focal onset.

Compliance

There is an expanding range of terms to describe the phenomenon whereby patients do not take their prescribed medication. Terms range from the old-fashioned (but well understood) 'compliance', the 1990s favourite 'adherence', through to the uber-PC 'concordance'. Whichever you prefer, it comes down to asking if patients (for what may in their minds be good reason) are taking the expected medication at the expected time at the expected dose. Most people recognise this as a problem in a significant minority of cases, and a few key questions can be useful when used sequentially (Table 2). If the patient describes difficulty sticking to the drug schedules, offering different regimens, differing timings or different formulations may help inspire his confidence in both you and the medication. Counselling about the negative effects of poorly controlled seizures may be appropriate, including a discussion about SUDEP. For some, reassurance about the lack of addictive or negative long-term effects will suffice.

Table 2 The compliance discussion.

* Do the drugs agree with you?

* Do you feel differently after you take them?

* Do you ever miss a dose to avoid these feelings?

Comorbidities – other effects of epilepsy

This term refers to the psychological and psychiatric phenomena that often accompany the diagnosis of epilepsy, usually in the form of depression and anxiety. Whether these are another marker of cerebral disease, a result of the psychological effects of seizures, or a side effect of AEDs is uncertain. It has been shown that patients with epilepsy and psychological and psychiatric comorbidity are less likely to go into remission, but the processes leading to resistance are poorly understood: whether these are both markers of a common cortical disease process or whether there are effects on compliance is also unknown.

Confounding lifestyle factors

Both sleep deprivation and alcohol play an important role in increasing the frequency of epileptiform discharges, especially in patients with an idiopathic generalised epilepsy. Discovery of such triggers is important, and again may lead to helpful discussion and counselling about the importance of avoidance. Recreational drug use is, among some age groups, an important consideration. Cannabis and opiates (including methadone) have less clearly defined proconvulsant effects, but their secondary effects on mood and compliance with 'proper' medicines may be important.

Consistency with the truth

Some patients may have a reason to exaggerate or inflate the number and / or severity of their seizures. These patients are (probably) rare, and the motivation may be financial (for DLA benefit, medicolegal reasons) or social (effects on family). Definitive diagnosis is difficult, but it is important to suspect this and to annotate it if necessary.

Management of poor drug response

If after addressing the above issues it becomes apparent that the patient has been genuinely refractory to their initial AED, then a full discussion must ensue. A revision of prognosis is important, and I would usually state that the chances of seizure freedom are now approximately 10%. The patient should be reminded that full control if not likely, is at least possible. The use of further investigation may be discussed at this point.

The rest of the discussion will focus on how drugs should be altered; the choice being between substitution or adding on. There is little trial evidence comparing these two approaches. There are reasons for preferring drug substitution, since this means patients will be on fewer treatments at any one time, with less expense, improved compliance, and less risk of pharmacodynamic or pharmacokinetic interactions. On the other hand, patients not responding to the first one or two drugs may benefit from a period of relative stability where you are changing only one thing at a time; phased substitution, i.e. adding on a drug with future expectation of withdrawal of baseline medication, is reasonable (particularly where care is taken to avoid mixing drugs with a tendency to interact). In the medium term a patient finding themselves free of seizures with add-on medication may be keen not to upset their new found control, and may dictate a slower pace of change!

The choice of second drug will depend on a number of factors (see below), the most important being the epilepsy classification (see Tables 3 and 4). Clinical trials have failed to demonstrate superiority of any particular agent, either in direct comparison or meta-analysis. The possibility of pharmacokinetic interactions, patient gender, side effects and possible side benefits will also be important.

Table 3 Drugs used in generalised epilepsies.

- Lamotrigine

- Topiramate

- Valproate

- Levetiracetam

- Carbamazepine (only with isolated generalised tonic-clonic seizures - can exacerbate myoclonus)

- Ethosuximide (only effective against childhood absence epilepsy)

Table 4 Drugs which can exacerbate generalised epilepsies.

- Carbamazepine

- Phenytoin

- Lamotrigine

- Gabapentin

- Pregabalin

Drug-drug interactions

We routinely accept that enzyme-inducing anti-epileptic drugs will require that add-on treatments are given at a higher dose. The most troublesome interaction of recent times between AEDs has been the use of lamotrigine alongside valproate, where inhibition of lamotrigine metabolism led to a marked increase in adverse effects.

It is vital that the possibility of OCP failure with traditional enzyme-inducing drugs or with higher doses of lamotrigine and topiramate should be remembered.

Patient gender

The use of drug combinations in pregnancy is to be avoided if at all possible. The safety of AEDs has undergone a great deal of work in recent years, those least likely to cause major malformations being carbamazepine and lamotrigine. While information on newer AEDs is sketchy, valproate should be avoided if at all possible. In some patients with IGE, valproate use may be inescapable, and in these circumstances the drug should be used at the lowest dose possible, acknowledging that the risk to the fetus of uncontrolled seizures may shift the risk / benefits towards use of such medications.

Drug side effects (and side benefits)

For some patients with pre-existing medical conditions, certain side effects are to be avoided. Specific conditions (e.g. nephrocalcinosis) may militate against single drugs, while others may make you keen to avoid specific adverse effects; for example, patients with hypertension, asthma, diabetes, or coronary heart disease may be made worse if they are subject to weight gain. Conversely, some medical conditions may respond to treatment with individual AEDs (see Table 5) or may benefit from side effects of individual AEDs (e.g. the above mentioned medical conditions and the potential benefits of drug-induced weight loss).

Table 5 Choosing the right drug - what may influence drug choice as mono and polypharmacy.

	Aggravate	Neutral	Help
Weight gain (hypertension, DM, etc)	Pregabalin Valproate Gabapentin ?Carbamazepine	Lamotrigine Levetiracetam Oxcarbazepine	Topiramate Zonisamide
Anxiety	Levetiracetam	Oxcarbazepine Valproate	Pregabalin ?Lamotrigine ?Carbamazepine
Depression	Topiramate ?Levetiracetam	Oxcarbazepine	Pregabalin ?Lamotrigine ?Carbamazepine
Migraine		Lamotrigine Oxcarbazepine	Topiramate Pregabalin Gabapentin Valproate

Management of continuing poor response

In a significant minority of patients, it will become apparent that even careful addition and manipulation of drugs will not be enough. In such cases, the neurologist is left trying to balance the best control possible for the individual patient with the fewest side effects.

It is important not to forget that surgical options may still be available, and that some patients with partial epilepsy may merit video telemetry to try and localise seizure origin, perhaps while reconsidering surgical intervention.

Surgical treatment of epilepsy

Two thirds of all patients with epilepsy will have seizures controlled by currently available AEDs. Even so, the chances of non-response are high enough after failure of the first two AEDs that surgical intervention should be considered at this point. In recent years there has been a gradual lowering of the threshold for epilepsy surgery, as the morbidity of seizures and the associated mortality (SUDEP) are increasingly recognized, but to justify any operation, the main question to be answered is whether the seizure disorder has a recognized focus that can be removed with little risk of neurological deficit or medical harm.

The success of epileptic surgery depends greatly on how well the epileptologist can define the area responsible for initiating the seizure discharges, the 'epileptogenic zone'. If this is identified, it becomes important to know whether its removal will cause any loss of function. In cases where complete resection is not possible, it may be reasonable to operate in the knowledge that only a partial resection is possible, the goal being to significantly reduce the seizure frequency or severity.

There are strict and established criteria for resective epilepsy surgery:

- ◆ confirmed diagnosis of epilepsy;
- ◆ medical intractability;
- ◆ resectable focus;

◆   motivated patient;
◆   no progressive underlying cause (e.g. Rasmussen's encephalitis).

The evaluation for epilepsy surgery is complex and requires a well-functioning, highly integrated multidisciplinary team, usually only found at tertiary medical centres. Assuming the diagnosis is secure, and that all of the ongoing attacks are clearly epileptic, non-invasive evaluation will suffice for epilepsy surgery consideration in 80-90% of patients. Concordance in findings (i.e. agreement from multiple testing on the site of seizure onset) predicts a good surgical outcome and allows one to proceed to surgery. If, however, the results tend to disagree, an invasive evaluation with depth electrodes may be considered. Invasive evaluation relies on more commitment from the patient and requires that there is a testable hypothesis of a resectable epileptogenic focus. Once the electrodes are in place, stimulation of electrodes can be used to delineate the eloquent cortex and avoid resection of or damage to the vital centres for fine movements, speech and / or memory.

Presurgical diagnostic evaluation includes:

◆   an accurate seizure description and a detailed patient history;
◆   EEG;
◆   video/EEG monitoring;
◆   neuro-imaging studies, e.g. MRI;
◆   functional imaging studies, e.g. PET/SPECT;
◆   neuropsychological evaluation.

Patient history

A detailed history should be taken of the progression of the epilepsy including the age of onset, any traumatic head injuries, CNS infections, in addition to detailed descriptions of seizures and if they have changed over time. Descriptions of seizures should again be obtained from a reliable witness, as the semiology of the predominant seizure pattern may yield clues to the site of origin of the epileptic activity. Previous AEDs and the patient's response to them should also be noted. A detailed review of all previous medical records should be obtained.

EEG

Where an attack is captured, EEG is the most specific method to define epileptogenic cortex. Both ictal and interictal recordings are of significance. If interictal spikes are consistent over time, they may be useful in confirming the epileptogenic area.

Video/EEG monitoring

Presurgical evaluation involves the patient spending time in the controlled environment of the Epilepsy Monitoring Unit (EMU). The EMU allows simultaneous video and EEG recordings via which seizures can be analyzed with the most precise accuracy. The 24-hour monitoring provides a safe environment for AEDs to be temporarily discontinued to encourage spontaneous seizures.

Surgical or invasive EEG

Often seizures arise from 'silent' cortex and ictal symptoms are only seen when the epileptic activity spreads to eloquent cortex; in such instances EEG may yield useful information in identifying the area of onset. Although surface EEG recordings are less sensitive than invasive studies, they provide the best overview of epileptic activity and approximation of the cortical area of seizure onset.

Invasive EEG techniques such as depth electrodes (see Figure 1), subdural strips and grids of electrodes have been developed. Such invasive EEG recordings are associated with additional risks, such as infection and haemorrhage, so undertaking these procedures requires some caution.

Neuro-imaging

Neuro-imaging studies as noted earlier can be divided into two categories: structural imaging and functional imaging.

Structural imaging studies provide information about any structural lesions and their anatomical relationship to the epileptogenic zone. Imaging is most likely to be important in TLE, but this concordance is poorer in extra-temporal epilepsies. Depending on the nature of the lesion

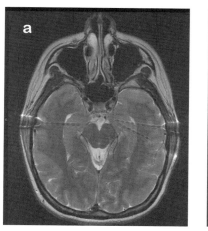
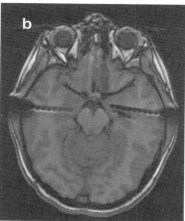
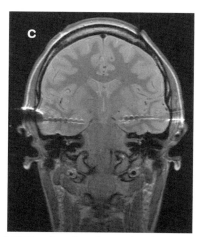

Figure 1 a) & b) Axial MRIs showing three depth electrodes (1 right, 2 left) to diagnose site of seizure onset. c) Coronal MRI showing depth electrodes.

and the degree of concordance with EEG findings, an invasive evaluation may be needed to further determine if the lesion alone or additional cortex should be surgically removed.

As techniques are refined, functional imaging is playing a more important role in the presurgical evaluation. Interictally, epileptogenic areas of cortex can be detected with [18F]fluorodeoxyglucose-PET. Ictal SPECT, however, is more reliable in showing regions of increased cerebral perfusion, especially in TLE. Functional MRI is also being used increasingly to help localize language in a non-invasive manner. As these advances continue, it may be used to test for sensory, motor and cognitive functions, yielding insight into the postoperative prognosis of these functions.

Neuropsychological evaluation

The importance of neuropsychological evaluation should not be dismissed; it plays an integral role providing valuable data on the patient's pre-operative cognitive abilities, which is used to counsel the patient on the cognitive risks associated with resective surgery and in planning post-surgical rehabilitation. Interpreting the results requires consideration of the sedating effect of any medication the patient is taking, as this may cause the appearance of under-performance. Similar impairments may be apparent if the patient has had a recent seizure.

Specific deficits may provide confirmatory information of the epileptogenic area's proximity to important structures. Patients with higher and lower IQs are at most risk to notice a decline in cognitive function after surgery, especially if the hippocampus of the dominant hemisphere is resected. An IQ below 70 is considered a poor prognostic factor for the preservation of baseline function, usually indicative of diffuse brain damage and a widespread epileptogenic area.

Status epilepticus (SE)

SE has been traditionally defined as a single clinical seizure lasting more than 30 minutes or repeated seizures over a period of time greater than 30 minutes without intervening recovery of consciousness. More importantly, it is a neurological emergency which needs immediate treatment. It is consistently under-recognized, despite its accompaniment by substantial morbidity and mortality. As very few seizures actually last longer than 5 minutes, it has been proposed that a patient who has a seizure that persists longer than 5 minutes should be considered in SE and treated accordingly.

Aetiology and clinical presentation

The incidence of SE is 20/100,000 per year in the general population; the highest incidence is in those aged 60 and over, followed by those under 12 months of age. The aetiologies of SE differ between different age groups. Febrile seizures or infections with fevers account for over half of all paediatric cases, while the leading aetiology among adults is cerebrovascular disease, including remote and acute stroke, and haemorrhage. In all age groups, lowered AEDs in treated patients with epilepsy accounted for a significant portion of the remaining cases. SE has a mortality rate between 3 and 40%, depending on age, aetiology, status type and duration. In addition, 10 to 23% of patients who survive SE are left with new or disabling neurological deficits, reinforcing the importance of prompt diagnosis and treatment. In 20% of cases, where SE is refractory to standard therapies, it is termed malignant status epilepticus, and refers to status that remains refractory to standard therapies and has a resultant poor prognosis.

The neurological examination can yield a variety of findings, and attention should be made not to overlook automatic movements or myoclonus. Where there is any suspicion of SE, an EEG should be done immediately. An EEG finding of continuous seizure activity is diagnostic of status epilepticus. The most important classification of SE involves the distinction between convulsive and non-convulsive SE (NCSE). Such classification is important as it is a major factor in determining morbidity and the aggressiveness of treatment, with more aggressive measures being taken with generalized tonic-clonic status. It is important to rule out other causes of cerebral dysfunction, such as hypoglycaemia, Korsakow syndrome or Herpes encephalitis. Once the airway has been secured and the patient is haemodynamically stable, they should be moved to the intensive care unit. Figure 2 depicts a recognized algorithm for the prompt and appropriate treatment of SE.

Convulsive SE

Convulsive SE can be easily identified through rhythmic jerking of the extremities at the onset. The history from any witnesses will make it clear that the intial manifestation of the event involved typical tonic-clonic seizure activity. Convulsive SE can be divided into two phases. The first phase consists of compensation, resulting from the massive release of catecholamines in response to the prolonged convulsion and causing an increase in heart rate, blood pressure and plasma glucose. Dangerous cardiac arrhythmias may be seen. As seizures continue there is a gradual rise in core body temperature (above 40°C), which may cause cerebral damage and is associated with a poor prognosis. Acidosis may develop as a result of increased lactic acid production, which in conjunction with a rise in CO_2 may result in a life-threatening narcosis. Increased autonomic activity is the hallmark of this phase. The homeostatic physiological mechanisms are initially able to compensate and maintain the blood-brain barrier and prevent cerebral damage.

The transition between phase one and two occurs approximately 30-60 minutes after the onset of continuous seizures, involving progressive decompensation, both systemic and cerebral, predisposing to severe cerebral damage. As autoregulation begins to fail, cerebral perfusion reduces as systemic blood pressure begins to fall. The high metabolic demands of seizing cortex cannot be met leaving it prone to ischaemia or metabolic damage and eventually in cerebral oedema. Systemically, the effects of prolonged convulsive SE include pulmonary hypertension and oedema, decreased cardiac output and eventually cardiac failure, as well as a wide variety of metabolic problems, e.g. disseminated intravascular coagulation and rhabdomyolysis. Later or milder manifestations may include automatic movements or myoclonus.

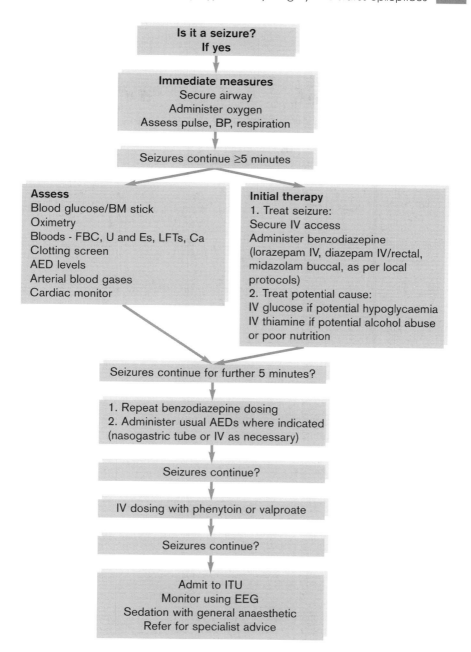

Figure 2 An algorithm for the prompt and appropriate treatment of SE.

Non-convulsive SE

This is sometimes known as partial status epilepticus. NCSE has a broad range of semiologies, some of which are very subtle and require a high level of suspicion from the physician to correctly identify NCSE (see Table 6). This explains the underdiagnosis of SE shown in several studies,

Table 6 Semiological spectrum of non-convulsive status epilepticus.

Positive symptoms	Negative symptoms
Aggression/agitation	Anorexia
Automatisms	Aphasia
Blinking	Amnesia
Delirium	Catatonia
Delusions	Coma
Echolalia	Lethargy
Facial twitching	Mutism
Laughing	Staring
Nausea/vomiting	
Nystagmus	
Perseveration	
Psychosis	
Tremulousness	
Weeping	

with as many as 34% of neurological ICU patients being reported to be in NCSE. As can be seen from the table, if the patient is not in convulsive status with generalized tonic-clonic movements, the reviewing physician needs a high level of suspicion. Factors raising this suspicion may be a marked variability in cognition, prolonged repeated automatisms, without other exacerbating factors such as infection or metabolic disturbance.

Pathophysiology of SE

Figure 3 shows the evolution of pathophysiologic changes during SE.

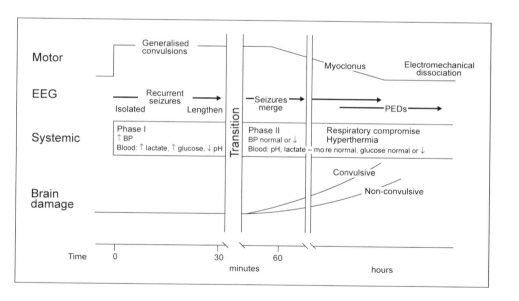

Figure 3 Metabolic and physiological changes of status epilepticus. BP = blood pressure; PEDs = periodic epileptiform discharges. *Reproduced with permission from Springer Science+Business Media. Robakis TK, Hirsch LJ. Literature review, case report, and expert discussion of prolonged refractory status epilepticus. Neurocrit Care 2006; 4(1): 35-46* [3].

Conclusions

Once epilepsy does not respond to the first drug, the choice of add-on or substitution treatment depends on a range of factors including other medication and other concomitant diseases.

In some ways, the profusion of new drugs has complicated an already difficult situation. There is no evidence to suggest that the number of patients who are seizure-free has reduced with increasing numbers of available AEDs. If not displaying enhanced efficacy, however, studies have shown that the newer drugs can offer improved tolerability. As always in medicine, the field of epileptology has shown progress by degrees. With time, we may have improved drugs offering universal seizure freedom, but until then we should learn to use the drugs we have already, and to guide our patients through the opportunities and limitations.

Surgical treatment for epilepsy is one of our success stories. Where patients are suitable, the seizure freedom rates are impressive and the morbidity is low. What is disappointing, is that we are having to work harder to identify the patients who will benefit from operation, and finding these patients to be increasingly scarce.

As the 20th century ended, it was hoped that digital EEG recording of prolonged spells, emergent functional imaging such as PET or spectroscopy, and increasingly sophisticated structural imaging would open the doors to curative surgery for more and more patients. In fact, most centres are seeing diminishing returns: the 'easy' temporal lobe resections have been done, and more and more work is going into identifying resectable lesions in decreasing numbers of patients with epilepsy. Most people would acknowledge that epilepsy surgery has become stuck: unless there is a dramatic shift in yield from better or more appropriate imaging, we will see fewer people undergoing resection in decades to come.

Status epilepticus is a medical emergency. Every acute physician should be equipped to deal with its varying presentations. Protocols for the immediate treatment of status epilepticus will vary between hospitals; the important aspects are to provide drugs to cut short seizure activity and to provide an environment where respiratory and cardiac function allow for oxygenation to be maintained.

Key Summary

◆ For the significant minority where things do not go well, there are a few key points.

◆ Make sure drug treatment is optimised.

◆ Make sure you think about whether an operation is going to be of benefit.

◆ Make sure you treat status epilepticus adequately aggressively.

References

1.   Kwan P, Brodie MJ. Early identification of refractory epilepsy. *N Engl J Med* 2000; 342: 314-9.
2.   Kanner AM. Psychiatric comorbidity in children with epilepsy. ... Or is it: epilepsy comorbidity in children with psychiatric disorders? *Epilepsy Currents* 2008; 8: 10-2.
3.   Robakis TK, Hirsch LJ. Literature review, case report, and expert discussion of prolonged refractory status epilepticus. *Neurocrit Care* 2006; 4(1): 35-46.

Chapter 12

Epilepsy at extremes of age

Epilepsy in children

As has been described, epilepsy is more common at the extremes of age, leaving relatively more children and adolescents affected by epilepsy. Many different epileptic syndromes occur during the first decade of life, and their correct and early diagnosis is important in allowing assessment of the child's overall and developmental prognosis.

It is important to remember that one type of seizure may arise from more than one epilepsy syndrome and as the child grows older seizure types may evolve. A thorough work-up is vital in ensuring an accurate diagnosis to help forewarn the patient and carers of the need for any future appropriate management. Diagnosis is not only based on seizure type but also on many other factors such as aetiology, neurologic examination and age of onset, in addition to EEG findings and neuro-imaging.

Aetiology

Most childhood epilepsies will have a genetic basis. Many hundreds of syndromes have been identified as having a strong association with epilepsy. In Table 1, we have divided diseases on whether they will come to the attention mainly of the neurologist (i.e. whether or not epilepsy is the sole or main manifestation). Further subdivision places them into monogenic conditions and polygenic conditions; these classes, of course, may be subject to change depending on the results of ongoing genetic studies.

Table 1 The most clinically common syndromes which have epilepsy as part of their spectrum.

Monogenic epilepsies

Channelopathies
- Autosomal dominant frontal lobe epilepsies

- Renal failure - action myoclonus syndrome

- Generalised epilepsy with febrile seizures plus

Malformations
- Gyral abnormalities - e.g. lissencephalopathy, polymicrogyria

- Heterotopias - e.g. subependymal nodular heterotopia, subcortical nodular heterotopia

- Gross malformations - e.g. megalencephaly, corpus callosum agenesis, microcephaly

- Cortical dysgenesis with neoplasia - e.g. dysembryoneuroepithelial tumour, hypothalamic hamartoma

- Other cortical dysplasia - e.g. focal cortical dysplasia

Monogenic syndromes with epilepsy as an accompanying or occasional manifestation

---

- Neurocutaneous syndromes - e.g. tuberous sclerosis, neurofibromatosis

- Metabolic syndromes - e.g. hexosaminidase deficiency, Niemann Pick disease, pyridoxine deficiency, sialidosis, mucopolysaccharidoses, Gaucher's disease

---

Chromosomal syndromes with epilepsy as an accompanying or occasional manifestation

---

- Ring 20 chromosome

- Down's syndrome

- Fragile X syndrome

- Klinefelter's syndrome

Polygenic pure epilepsies

- Idiopathic generalised epilepsies - e.g. juvenile myoclonic epilepsy, childhood absence epilepsy

---

It should be noted that the monogenic conditions are almost exclusively channelopathies, although again, future work may expand the remit of these culprit genes.

In children, as in adults, the idiopathic epilepsies have an anatomically normal brain and a neurological examination without any significant findings. There tends to be a familial pattern with a typical age at onset and it is generally believed that they are due to specific genetic abnormalities (some as yet undefined). With the advancements of molecular biology in the last 25 years, there has been a huge increase in the understanding of idiopathic epilepsies, many being reclassified as genetic once the specific culprit mutation has been identified.

Many of the abnormalities involve the genes for ion channels, with each specific ion channel being associated (though not exclusively) with different syndromes. Culprit mutations have been found in genes for channels of sodium, potassium, chloride, and calcium.

Structural and metabolic causes of epilepsy are also prone to occur in childhood, arising from inherited disorders of metabolism, birth injury (i.e. probably ischaemic) and congenital malformations. Trauma and neoplasms are also important to consider in childhood and adolescence; the onset of seizures, however, may occur soon after the insult or be delayed for many years.

Febrile seizures

Although febrile seizures are classified as 'provoked seizures', their frequency and their long-term effects make it important to have these discussed at this point. Febrile convulsions are the most common type of seizure in infancy seen by physicians in emergency departments. They are a cause of concern for both parents and medical providers alike, usually occurring within 24 hours of a fever greater than 38.5°C. Approximately 2-5% of Caucasian infants and 6-9% of Japanese infants are affected by febrile seizures. Febrile seizures are classified as either simple or complex, by virtue of their severity (Table 2) and their propensity to cause or be

Table 2 Differentiation of simple and complex febrile convulsions.

	Simple febrile seizures	Complex febrile seizures
Age at occurrence	6 months - 6 years	6 months or 5 years
Seizure type	Generalized tonic-clonic No focal features	Partial seizure Focal features such as involvement of one side of body
Duration	<10 minutes	$\geq$15 minutes
Reoccurrence	None in 24 hours	Recurring within 24 hours
Previous neurological problem	No	Yes/No

associated with long-term neurological complications and resultant epilepsy.

Simple febrile seizures have an excellent prognosis, usually with no evidence of a prior CNS insult or anomaly. Physical examination and EEG are normal, but there is often a family history of febrile seizures. The low recurrence risk for simple febrile convulsions means that most children with febrile seizures do not need to receive anti-epileptic drugs.

If the first febrile seizure occurs before the age of 1, there is a recurrence rate of 50%. If the seizure occurs after one year the recurrence rate is 25%. Eighty-eight percent of recurrences occur within 2 years of the first seizure. Factors known to increase the risk of recurrence include complex febrile seizures, the presence of prior abnormal neurologic or developmental status prior to the febrile seizure, and a history of unprovoked seizures in a first-degree relative. However, if the child has prolonged convulsions or frequent recurrences, treatment should be considered including intermittent rectal diazepam, or daily treatment with standard anti-epileptic drugs.

There are changes at several genetic loci currently identified as responsible for febrile seizures. The presence of these genetic changes is increasingly recognised as underlying the complex or recurrent febrile convulsions, as well as those occurring at a later age, as in for example, generalized epilepsy with febrile seizures plus (GEFS+). This syndrome results from a wide variety of genetic mutations and presents with a wide range of phenotypes even within the same family, from atypical febrile seizures (continuing beyond 6 years of age) to severe myoclonic epilepsy of infancy (SMEI). Mutations in genes for sodium channels and $GABA_A$ receptor subunit genes have been identified in GEFS+.

Common childhood syndromes

Benign focal epilepsy with centrotemporal spikes

This used to be known as rolandic epilepsy, and is a common type of idiopathic, localization-related epilepsy. The peak incidence occurs between 8 to 10 years of age, but it may arise anytime between 4 to 12 years of age. This syndrome consists of infrequent largely nocturnal (80% are solely nocturnal) partial motor seizures of the face and arm or generalized tonic-clonic seizures. The EEG shows a distinctive sharp wave abnormality over the centrotemporal region, most marked during sleep. Usually these children have normal neurologic examinations and their brains have normal anatomic architecture. In most cases medication is not needed; however, a good response may be obtained in most children with carbamazepine or gabapentin. It is important to identify children in this group, as the family can be reassured that their child should have spontaneous remission of their seizures by the age of 16 years.

Childhood and juvenile absence epilepsy

Childhood absence epilepsy (this is the syndrome originally named 'petit mal') is a form of idiopathic, generalized epilepsy. It usually presents at 6 or 7 years of age, always involving brief absences and occasionally (around 50%) involving generalized tonic-clonic seizures. A characteristic 3Hz spike and slow wave complex pattern is seen on EEG, especially during hyperventilation. Patients usually respond well to anti-epileptic medication and seizures usually remit spontaneously before early adulthood.

Juvenile absence epilepsy has similar clinical and electrophysiologic presentations, but the peak age of presentation is at 12 years. Patients, however, are more likely (80%) to have generalized tonic-clonic seizures. Absence status may be easily overlooked, presenting as a prolonged, subtle episode of confusion and unusual behaviour. AEDs are usually effective, although the long-term evolution of juvenile absence epilepsy is unclear.

Juvenile myoclonic epilepsy

Juvenile myoclonic epilepsy presents most frequently in adolescence with a combination of myoclonic and generalised tonic-clonic seizures. Anyone with recent onset of generalised tonic-clonic seizures should be asked about the prior incidence of myoclonic jerks as they may not have been severe or sustained enough to merit seeking medical attention. Seizures in these patients are particularly prone to exacerbation by sleep deprivation or alcohol use. While lifelong treatment is usually necessary, the seizures usually respond well to reasonable doses of broad-spectrum anti-epileptic drugs.

Epilepsy in the elderly

As the general population ages, the increased occurrence of epilepsy in elderly patients becomes an increasingly important public health problem. There remains a misperception that epilepsy does not affect older patients - one recent study showed that the ultimately correct diagnosis of epilepsy was considered in only 73.3% of cases by an internist or primary care physician during the initial evaluation. The differential diagnosis of new-onset seizures in the elderly can be complicated by the physiologic changes of aging in addition to the concurrence of other pathological states; however, greater awareness of epilepsy - its frequency, morbidity and mortality - is necessary amongst those who care for elderly patients.

The incidence of unprovoked seizures increases with age and is greatest for those over 75 years of age. A significantly higher mortality is associated with these seizures in comparison to younger age groups, and there is a higher mortality risk from status epilepticus. Notwithstanding the frequent co-occurrence of confounding and confusing comorbidities, a correct diagnosis is made more difficult, as epilepsy may have slightly different manifestations compared to younger patients. Cerebrovascular disease has been identified as the most common aetiology for seizures in the elderly, followed by degenerative diseases and trauma; neoplasms account for a much smaller fraction of seizures. Cerebral infarction alone can increase the risk of late-onset seizures up to 23 times that of the general public. The majority of elderly patients with epilepsy will have risk factors such as dyslipidemia (80%), cardiovascular disease or hypertension (66%) and diabetes (28%).

The classic clinical picture of a generalized tonic-clonic seizure associated with epilepsy is less common among the elderly. The more frequent focal neurologic symptoms may be attributed to other 'geriatric' pathologies such as transient ischaemic attacks (TIAs). While both will have initial focal neurological symptoms, seizures may be differentiated by ictal and post-ictal global disturbances causing confusion or altered mental state. The post-ictal period in the elderly, unlike in younger adults, can last from hours to 1-2 weeks. Of course, attribution of cognitive impairment requires exclusion of other causes such as adverse effects of medication, infection, dehydration, low-output cardiac syndromes, metabolic disturbances, migraine and sleep disorders. Just to confuse things further, seizures in the elderly may take slightly different forms than in younger patients. Table 3 shows how we must broaden the possible range of 'normal' manifestations in the elderly.

Investigation may be more complicated in the elderly. If the EEG should be treated with caution in adults, it should be treated with even more caution at the extremes of age: children and the elderly are more likely to show focal and generalised changes where there have been no seizures. A finding of 'focal slowing' on EEG may lead the unwary to forget the wide range of conditions that can cause this, and misattribute any symptoms to epilepsy. The importance of recording a typical event (see section on EEG in Chapter 7) is even more marked in the elderly.

The relationship between dose and serum level of AEDs can vary greatly in the elderly due to the physiologic changes that occur with aging. As albumin concentrations decrease, the protein binding capacity also

Table 3 Clinical presentation of complex partial seizures.

	18 - 65 years	>65 years
Most common seizure focus	Temporal lobe	Extratemporal lobe
Aura	Common Specific manifestation e.g. epigastric, etc.	Less common Non-specific manifestation e.g. dizziness
Motor manifestations	Occasional complex motor e.g. behavioural arrest $\rightarrow$ automatisms	Occasional simple motor e.g. behavioural arrest $\rightarrow$ clonus of one limb
Secondary generalization	Common	Less common
Post-ictal state	Very brief: 5-15 minutes	Long: Hours - weeks

decreases. AED clearance reduces with lower glomerular filtration rates and lower hepatic capacity. The volume of distribution for lipid-soluble drugs usually increases with age. As a result, the half-life of many AEDs is longer in the elderly than in young adults. Most elderly patients are the recipients of polypharmacy due to multiple comorbidities that may lead to undesirable interactions with AEDs, meaning that the advantages of AED monotherapy in the elderly are even greater.

The elderly are more susceptible to the neurological side effects of AEDs, and the treating doctor should remain alert to the possibility of confusion, general ill health, changes in mood, uncharacteristic motor or behavioural disturbances.

The picture is not entirely without hope: epilepsy in the elderly often benefits from greater responsiveness to lower doses of AEDs. Treatment in the elderly, therefore, should utilise low doses of the best tolerated medications which have fewest pharmacokinetic interactions and variations. As a general rule, therapeutic regimes should be started at lower doses and slowly increased in an incremental fashion. Hepatic and renal function may need to be monitored with enzyme-inducing drugs, and some may advocate measuring AED plasma levels if new clinical symptoms emerge. Table 4 lists the most common side effects associated with the most commonly prescribed AEDs.

Table 4 Clinical caveats and side effects associated with commonly used AEDs.

AED	Hepatic impairment	Renal impairment	Neurologic side effects	Systemic side effects	Other
Carbamazepine			Impaired gait Tremor	Hyponatraemia Drug-induced osteoporosis Promotes arrhythmias Hypotension	Urinary retention Caution with diabetes
Gabapentin		Reduce dose	Sedation		
Lamotrigine	Reduce dose			Promotes arrhythmias Hypotension	Interacts with other AEDs
Levetiracetam		Reduce dose	Sedation /agitation		
Phenobarbital		Reduce dose	Ataxia Lethargy Behavioural changes		Drug-induced osteoporosis Sedation with benzodiazepines
Phenytoin	Reduce dose		Ataxia Sedation Neuropathy	Promotes arrhythmias Hypotension	Drug-induced osteoporosis Caution with diabetes
Topiramate	Reduce dose	Reduce dose	Confusion Tremor		Renal stones
Valproate	Reduce dose		Encephalopathy	Easy bruising	

The presence of comorbidities which complicate epilepsy and lead to risk may make treatment and prognosis difficult. The co-occurrence of seizures and osteoporosis may explain the two-fold increase in risk of fractures in elderly patients with epilepsy. This is made worse by the decrease in bone mineral density associated with the chronic use of certain AEDs. Some doctors used to advocate bone health assessment is carried out on a regular basis, in addition to calcium supplementation.

There is a higher incidence of depression among the elderly with epilepsy in comparison to others of the same age. There are many possible reasons for this, ranging from the neurochemical changes wrought by seizures, to anxiety about seizures and their consequences, and primary effects of anti-epileptic medications. Features of clinical depression should always be sought, and lead to appropriate medication which will help both the mood disorder and therefore increase chances of seizure control. Measures such as provision of a personal alarm can be very useful for both the patient and family, giving both confidence and assurance that help will arrive during a seizure.

Conclusions

In summary, epilepsy in childhood has subtle differences to that seen in adults. When genetic or developmental syndromes are excluded, response rates tend to be higher, and the prospect of long-term AED withdrawal is correspondingly raised.

Epilepsy in the elderly is becoming increasingly recognised. The good news is this usually responds better - often to low doses of well-tolerated anti-epileptic drugs. It is important to reassure the elderly patient that the recent onset of seizures does not usually indicate a tumour, dementia, or another psychiatric disorder. We would stress the high response rates in elderly patients, and the wide range of medications available. Careful thought to regimes and social support may lead to a more rapid return to normal life uninhibited by seizures. Care usually involves a multi-disciplinary team with important input from social services, and remedial and occupational therapists.

Key Summary

◆ Epilepsy is as common in the elderly as in children.

◆ There are probably different mechanisms underlying the epilepsies in these two age groups.

◆ Epilepsy in the elderly usually responds well to treatment - often at a low dose.

◆ Epilepsy is more likely to undergo remission with time in children and allow treatment withdrawal.

References

1. Lueders HO, Noachtar S. *Epileptic Seizures: Pathophysiology and Clinical Semiology*, 1st ed. New York: Churchill Livingstone, 2000.
2. Shorvon SD. *Handbook of Epilepsy Treatment: Forms, Causes and Therapy in Children and Adults*, 2nd ed. Oxford: Blackwell Science, 2005.
3. Kotagal P, Lueders HO. *The Epilepsies: Etiologies and Prevention*. San Diego: Academic Press, 1999.
4. Lueders HO. *Epilepsy Surgery*. New York: Raven Press, 1992.
5. Engle Jr. J, Pedley TA, Aicardi J, *et al. Epilepsy: a Comprehensive Textbook*. Philadelphia: Lippincott Williams & Wilkins, 1999.
6. Hauser WA, Annegers JF, Kurland LT. Incidence of epilepsy and unprovoked seizures in Rochester, Minnesota: 1935-1984. *Epilepsia* 1993; 34(3): 453-68.
7. Brodie MJ, Elder AT, Kwan P. Epilepsy in later life. *Lancet Neurol* 2009; 8(11): 1019-30.
8. Wyllie E, Gupta A, Lachhwani DK. *The Treatment of Epilepsy: Principles and Practice*. Philadelphia: Lippincott Williams & Wilkins, 2005.

Chapter 13
Specific situations

Women with epilepsy

The care of women with epilepsy should involve a multidisciplinary team to accurately assess and pre-empt risks specific to women, whether through the epileptic process or its treatment. Special considerations regarding treatment decisions must be made in conjunction with the different reproductive stages of a woman's life.

Menstruation

Oestrogen is known to lower seizure threshold and increase seizure susceptibility, while progesterone has opposite effects. Almost 25% of women with epilepsy report seizure patterns associated with their menstrual cycle, although closely monitored seizure diaries often fail to provide a specific pattern. With hormonal fluctuations it could be seen that the marked rise in oestrogen prior to ovulation or drop in progesterone could potentially alter seizure threshold.

Catamenial epilepsy should be defined as a doubling of the baseline seizure frequency during hormonal changes in the menstrual cycle. Using this defintion, it becomes apparent that this is rarer than many women believe.

Three patterns have been identified:

◆ C1: during perimenstrual days;
◆ C2: at ovulation;
◆ C3: in the setting of anovulation when the luteal phase is inadequate.

All female patients should use a monthly calendar to record both seizures and menstrual flow for the evaluation of menstrual seizure patterns. In our experience, changing hormonal patterns proves disappointing in controlling seizures unless there is a well-defined catamenial pattern as demonstrated by reliable seizure diaries.

Fertility

Women with epilepsy experience reduced fertility in comparison to the general population. This may relate to epileptic discharges disrupting the hypothalamic and hypophyseal function and causing increased anovulatory cycles in women with epilepsy. Irregular menstrual cycles and polycystic ovary syndrome are also common. Clinicians should be sensitive to any evidence of irregular menstruation or other hormonal imbalances, such as obesity or hirsuitism, and ensure that such women undergo further evaluation with a gynaecologist to minimize the long-term health risks.

Contraception

Discussion of hormonal contraceptives should take place at an early stage (in fact early and often!) with appropriate encouragement for concomitant barrier methods where necessary. It is vital for clinicians to know which AEDs cause a significant drop in anti-contraceptive levels of oestrogen. Table 1 lists the most common AEDs and their effect on hormonal contraceptives.

Where AED-related enzyme induction occurs, measures should bolster contraceptive efficacy. Solutions include prescribing contraceptives with a higher oestrogen content, a gestagen-releasing intra-uterine device or quarterly injections of medroxyprogesterone acetate. The last may have

Table 1 Effect of AEDs on hormonal contraceptives.

Enzyme-inducing AEDs (reduce contraceptive effects)	Enzyme-inhibiting AEDs (no effect on contraceptive effect)	AEDs without an effect on contraceptive efficacy or pharmacokinetics
Carbamazepine	Felbamate	Ethosuximide
Oxcarbamazepine	Valproate	Gabapentin
Phenobarbital		Lamotrigine
Phenytoin		Levetiracetam
Topiramate >200mg/day		Tiagabine
		Zonisamide

benefits in reducing catamenial seizures. There is a lack of evidence on the usefulness or otherwise in women with epilepsy of intravaginal rings which release low doses of oestrogen.

Pregnancy

Much has been written about this topic, but it is important to contextualise the medical angst that has taken root over the last 20 years or so. Patients should realise that over 90% of women with epilepsy have uncomplicated pregnancies and healthy children. Epilepsy and its treatment may cause slight increases in vaginal bleeding, hyperemesis gravidarum and pre-eclampsia in women with epilepsy. Women who smoke are advised to stop, as they are at an increased risk for premature contractions, premature labour and delivery. Previous seizure freedom (for more than 9 months) prior to pregnancy is unlikely to be disrupted during pregnancy.

Seizure freedom is the goal during pregnancy, since as well as maternal injury there is the threat to the fetus of induction of hypoxia, acidosis and blunt trauma, all of which increase the risk for developmental problems, stillbirth or spontaneous abortion. Through understandable concern about the risk of AED treatment, women often stop or reduce their AEDs without medical consultation. To avert this where possible, it should be made clear that the risks to the fetus during tonic-clonic seizures outweigh the risks of AED exposure. Where poor adherence is thought to be a problem, free and total drug levels should be measured monthly.

Table 2 lists the teratogenic properties of the most commonly prescribed AEDs and the risk level attributed by the FDA. Pregnancy registers will provide increasingly valuable information about the relative dangers of AEDs, but there remain important questions about the long-term effects on performance IQ from pre-natal exposure to AEDs.

Table 2 Teratogenic properties of common AEDs.

AED	Major malformations	FDA pregnancy category
Carbamazepine	Spina bifida, craniofacial and cardiac defects	D
Ethosuximide	No specific	C
Gabapentin	Unknown	C
Lamotrigine	Cleft palate, major congenital malformation	C
Levetiracetam	No specific	C
Oxcarbamazepine	No specific	C
Phenobarbital	Cleft palate, cardiac defects	D
Phenytoin	Cleft palate, cardiac defects	D
Tiagabine	No specific	C
Topiramate	No specific	C
Valproate	Spina bifida, craniofacial and skeletal defects	D
Zonisamide	No specific	C

Efficacy of AEDs may be affected during pregnancy. Physiological changes such as altered gastrointestinal motility, an increase in plasma volume and changes in liver function and protein binding, alter drug metabolism and may reduce the total serum concentrations of most AEDs. Therefore, treatment should be individually tailored for each patient.

Management of epilepsy with pregnancy should ideally begin before conception. The patient should be encouraged to optimise seizure control and reinforce the importance of folate supplementation. As with the general population, low maternal folic acid levels are associated with fetal neural tube defects. Some AEDs, such as valproate and carbamazepine, may lower folic acid levels. Despite a lack of specific evidence, there is a strong argument that all patients of child-bearing age should be on a long-term daily folic acid supplement (4-5mg/day). This replacement should continue at least until the end of the first trimester.

Once conception is achieved, the patient should average one consultation with a neurologist each trimester and 6-8 weeks after delivery. Most obstetricians perform early ultrasonography at 12 weeks and measure maternal alpha fetoprotein at 16 weeks. A more detailed anatomic ultrasonography should be performed at 16-18 weeks and repeated at 22 weeks (if needed) to detect neural tube defects, as well as craniofacial, cardiac and skeletal malformations of the fetus. If there are specific clinical indications, amniocentesis and other specific tests should be performed as the obstetrician deems necessary.

In the run-up to delivery, women on enzyme-inducing AEDs are also advised to take a vitamin K supplement (10mg/day) during the last 4 weeks of pregnancy to help prevent haemorrhagic syndrome in the infant, resulting from a deficiency of vitamin K-dependent clotting factors. In the event of such a haemorrhage, prompt intravenous administration of fresh frozen plasma is essential.

Delivery and postnatal period

The risk of seizures occurring during delivery is small (under 5%) and tends to occur in women who have had frequent seizures during pregnancy. Many women with epilepsy are concerned about such an occurrence and its ramifications, and great emphasis should be put on planning the delivery and, if necessary, counselling. Epilepsy *per se* is not an indication for Caesarean section. Women and their birth partners should be advised to bring their own anti-epileptic medication, to ensure a continuous and routine supply on maternity wards. As far as possible, hyperventilation and exhaustion should be avoided. If emergency treatment of seizures is required, benzodiazepines should be used. It is important to exclude the onset of eclampsia and, if necessary, commence treatment with magnesium sulfate.

The metabolism of AEDs by the fetus is limited and the infant's AED level will decrease in the days following delivery. A withdrawal syndrome may be seen with older drugs such as phenobarbital, phenytoin and benzodiazepines. This will render the neonate lethargic, irritable and difficult to feed.

Concerns about infant exposure to AEDs should not deter mothers from breastfeeding (they will have had plenty of exposure in the previous 9 months anyway!). AEDs are excreted in breast milk in inverse proportion to their protein binding. Maternal pharmacokinetics will return to normal prepregnancy levels within 10 to 14 days postpartum, requiring re-adjustment of AEDs to pre-pregnancy doses to prevent toxicity. Where considered appropriate, AED levels could be measured at 1 and 3 days, and 2 weeks postpartum.

The intial postpartum period is both exciting and worrying for any woman, and the potential for seizures should not be allowed to spoil this. Simple advice and measures (see Table 3) may give confidence and reassurance for women who continue to experience seizures or worries about seizures.

Menopause

The effects of menopause on epilepsy are variable and there is an even split among women experiencing a deterioration, improvement, or static

Table 3 Tips for new mothers with epilepsy.

- Take your medication at regular intervals, despite disrupted routines

- Minimize sleep deprivation
  - Sleep when the baby sleeps
  - If breast feeding: have someone bring the baby to you for night feedings
  - If bottle feeding: have someone else do night feedings

- Baby should not sleep in bed with you

- Change diapers with baby in a safe position, e.g. in the crib

- Only bathe the baby when someone else is there to help

- When transporting the baby, strap them in a stroller to prevent drop injuries

---

seizure control. In keeping with an increased incidence of menstrual irregularities, an earlier onset of menopause is also associated with epilepsy.

Perimenopausal cyclic irregularities can increase seizure frequency, thought to be associated with fluctuating levels of oestrogen and progesterone. There are conflicting data on the usefulness of oestrogen substitution (hormone replacement therapy [HRT]) on seizure frequency, and it is not standard to provide this for the purposes of improving seizure control.

Osteoporosis

Several AEDs are associated with various disturbances in bone metabolism, particularly those with a tendency to induce hepatic enzymes (see Table 4), and the diagnosis of epilepsy leaves both sexes at risk of early development of osteoporosis. This risk is, however, greatest in postmenopausal women.

Table 4 Bone metabolism abnormalities associated with AEDs.

Biochemical marker	Effect measured in serum
Calcium	Decrease
Phosphate	Decrease
Alkaline phosphatase	Increase
Vitamin D metabolites	Decrease
Markers of bone formation	Increase
Markers of bone resorption	Increase

The additional threat of trauma due to seizures and falls (caused by AED-induced dizziness and ataxia) make it important to educate women about the risk factors for osteoporosis and the benefits of early treatment. It has been recommended that all women should undergo a bone density measurement (using dual energy X-ray absorption [DXA]) 5 years after initiation of AED treatment, and on commencement of treatment in postmenopausal women. DXA scans should be repeated every 2 years, to detect metabolic disturbances early. The benefits of calcium and vitamin D supplementation as well as weight-bearing exercise should be stressed.

Single seizure

The patient with a single seizure firstly involves a diagnostic challenge. Usually, the patient with a blackout will present to emergency services. The first job of medical staff attending is to make sure that the culprit event has passed. If the event continues, then the patient by definition is in status epilepticus and the management is as already described.

If (as is usual) the event has passed, the main task is to get a history from the patient and, if possible, at least one eye witness. If this can be done while events are fresh in everyone's mind, then there is a better chance of making a real estimate of timing and sequence order. The nature of information needed is listed in Chapter 7 on diagnosis. It may in fact be reasonable (and may be better) to get this information after a few days.

About the only advantage of living in the age of mobile communications is that we can get a useful description from the checkout girl at Marks and Spencer. If a diagnosis of seizure is made, an examination may show up signs of neurological deficit (remembering that cognitive difficulties represent a neurological deficit). Should such signs be present, then the patient merits urgent imaging studies (MRI or CT of the brain depending on local availability) before discharge home. Most centres persist in checking FBC and U & Es, but the yield in otherwise healthy adults is very small and I would doubt that these in themselves should delay discharge.

Where neurological state has returned to normal, the patient should be referred to a local first seizure clinic or neurology clinic. UK guidelines have stressed that such review should be available within 2 weeks, but it is only now that it is becoming achievable. The first seizure clinic visit is important, as it gives a chance for checking the diagnosis. As shown, many patients will have simply fainted, and the referring doctor will be 'just checking' by referring for a neurological review, particularly where they have felt uneasy in attributing jerking or urinary incontinence to syncope.

Once the diagnosis of seizure has been made, the doctor has two questions to answer:

◆   why should this patient have a seizure (see Table 5)?; and
◆   are there any seizures going on that are so far undetected (see Table 6)?

An important aspect of the visit is to dispense occupational, sporting, and driving advice. These are often dealt with poorly (if at all!) by primary care and emergency doctors, and it is vital that someone discusses these with patients as early as possible. Avoidance of situations where the patient or others are at risk is paramount.

Table 5 Why should this patient have seizures or epilepsy?

Genetics	Family history of faints, fits, drop attacks, or seizures. (also picks up on cardiac problems)
Birth injury	Were you premature, a 'blue baby', or born by emergency Caesarean section?
Congenital problems	Did you walk and talk at the correct stage when you were young?
Febrile convulsions	Did you ever have any fever fits or febrile convulsions when you were a young child?
Head injury	Have you ever had any skull fractures or knocked yourself out for minutes or been concussed for hours?
Infections	Ever had any meningitis or encephalitis?
Brain insult	Have any history of strokes or TIAs?
Alcohol	Regularly drink? How many units per week?
Drugs	Have any history of exposure to street drugs?

Table 6 Are there any other seizures that have not yet been picked up?

Nocturnal GTC	Have you ever woken in the morning having bitten your tongue, wet the bed, fallen out of bed, or injured yourself?
Myoclonus	Have you ever had any jerking movements of the arms or legs when you are up and about in the morning?
Complex partial seizures	Have you ever had any episodes of lost time, blank spells, odd behaviour or automatic behaviour, or episodes where people said you would not respond to them? (The mention of 'odd behaviour' usually gets a wry smile. Get used to it, and enjoy it! NB - ignoring your spouse when there's a newspaper in the room is physiological)
Absences	Have you ever had any episodes of blank staring spells?
Photosensitivity	Have you ever been made to feel unwell by flashing or flickering lights? (e.g. stroboscopic lights, light through railings, trees while walking or driving)

Counselling is also a good part of the clinic visit. Relatives will be worried about recurrence risk and, in particular, the risk of SUDEP. This will rarely be articulated, and it is best if this can be introduced largely to emphasise how low the risk is in most patients.

The sense of loss of control is often overwhelming; it is the doctor's job to address this in a positive way, emphasising the recurrence risk of around 40%, and the importance of investigations for prognostic rather than diagnostic reasons (see Table 7).

Table 7 Relative risk of recurrence after a single seizure.

Risk factor for recurrence of seizure	1 - Major brain injury	2 - Abnormality on imaging	3 - Epileptiform abnormality on EEG
	0/3 Recurrence risk = 20%	1/3 Recurrence risk = 40%	2/3 (including abnormal EEG) Recurrence risk = 60%

Treatment of single seizure

The tendency to provide treatment after a single documented seizure is something that varies widely between countries. The MESS study showed that long-term prognosis is not helped by the provision of AED treatment after a single seizure. There is no decrease in mortality, and no evidence of increasing frequency of refractory epilepsy where treatment is withheld until the development of further episodes.

Where the recurrence risk is higher than 50% (see Table 7), then the chances of having a further seizure is similar to the chances in someone who has experienced two unprovoked seizures. Treatment with an appropriate AED can then be justified.

Patients with learning difficulties

It is not within the scope of this book to examine the myriad syndromes that can cause learning difficulties and epilepsy among neurological problems. Adult neurologists and primary care physicians have a particular set of duties when they are 'inheriting' such patients from paediatrician colleagues, but syndromic diagnosis is not usually prominent among them.

By the time the patients arrive for their first visit to the adult clinic, they will already have undergone both imaging and EEG to try and establish not just their epilepsy syndrome, but the underlying genetic and pathological reasons for their disorders. On the assumption that this has been done to everyone's satisfaction, the clinician who simply deals with seizures has the slightly less daunting task of planning any future interventions and making the most of the patient's existing function.

If the syndromic diagnosis is not clear, then further investigation with imaging and EEG may help provide an insight into any specific treatments that may help. A number of causes of learning difficulty should have been excluded or at least considered (see Table 8), and if this is not the case, then reassessment by geneticists or metabolic specialists may have to be considered. If the syndromic diagnosis is clear, and previous treatment has been adequate, it will probably have occurred to the family and carers that the chances of seizure freedom, or of a 'cure' are negligible.

In order to direct the need for further treatment, there are some questions that need to be asked when you encounter a patient for the first time - some of which may be familiar!

Is the patient having seizures?

I'm sorry if this is repetitive, but it is vital to ask. Carers and doctors can sometimes be guilty of tramline thinking; that since the patient has epilepsy, any change in behaviour is a result of further seizures. In fact, patients with learning difficulties are at risk of other causes of attack; behavioural changes may arise as a result of any worries, uncertainty or social upheaval, gastro-oesophageal reflux, or other undiagnosed painful

Table 8 Genetic causes of learning difficulty and epilepsy.

Condition	Summary	Nature of epilepsy, provisional
Angelman syndrome	Autosomal recessive condition with characteristic EEG changes and epilepsy. Phenotype classically 'happy puppet' appearance and behaviour	Seizure onset in early childhood, evolution of seizure type from high-voltage slow bursts in infancy to diffuse spike and wave in middle childhood. Atypical absences and absence status
Tuberous sclerosis	Genetic abnormality usually on short arm of chromosome 15 affecting GABA receptors. Cortical malformations and epilepsy will result from this. Characteristic skin changes of epiloia, shagreen patch	62% risk of developing seizures
Fragile X syndrome	Chromosomal changes in X chromosome	Debate over specific EEG changes similar to benign childhood epilepsy with centro-temporal spikes
Down's syndrome	Trisomy of chromosome 23. Degenerative changes in brain cause generalised EEG changes in older patients with myoclonus and generalised tonic-clonic seizures	Seizure prevalence of 1-13% Two peak incidences in first year of life and later life, the latter being associated with the presence of Alzheimer's disease

or uncomfortable conditions. Patients with learning difficulties are at as much risk of cardiac difficulties as anyone else. Mortality from syncope will in fact be increased in those with congenital cardiac abnormalities.

Are these seizures a threat to life?

Presentation of a crowded seizure diary can leave the clinician searching for alternative or additional drug therapies. If the episodes are not endangering the patient, if, for example, episodes are short-lived with no cyanosis or repeated injury, then the family may be reassured that there is no need to rush into a decision on treatment changes. Of course, clinicians and families of those with learning difficulty should be aware that frequent prolonged generalised tonic-clonic seizures (to which patients with severe cortical disease may be more prone) are a risk factor for SUDEP. It is important that such discussions take place to forewarn and inform families and carers, but also to place the risks in context. The place of rescue medication should be clarified.

Are these episodes a threat to quality of life?

Even if episodes of seizure are not dangerous, they may be frequent enough to disrupt the patient's daily activities, whether they are disabled or prevented from taking part in clubs and placements because of post-ictal incapacity or for preventative reasons. Even if seizures are not hazardous, their social consequences may be enough to justify more aggressive medication. You might not want to think that patients should undergo increasing medication for the convenience of carers, but no-one can underestimate the difficulties caused by having to care for someone with frequent falls or wandering episodes.

Is the existing medication causing or likely to cause side effects?

Behavioural changes caused by AEDs are not uncommon, and should always be considered where a patient becomes more depressed or anxious following treatment change. The 'normal' behaviour for a particular patient may in fact be a sedated version of the real thing, and it is recognised that some 'agitating' AEDs are in fact merely non-sedating, allowing the 'real' patient to emerge, however inconvenient and trying this may be. Those with mild learning difficulty may still have child-bearing potential, and changing to an AED with a safer profile in any potential pregnancy may be in the patient's interest.

Are there any medications that may help?

Choosing medications for patients with learning difficulties involves the same trade-off as with other patients. The clinician has to decide if other medication would be more liable to reduce seizures than cause more side effects. Severe recurrent life-threatening seizures may require medications which necessitate more intensive monitoring such as stiripentol, vigabatrin, bromides, or felbamate.

Pseudoseizures

It has long been recognised in many cultures that humans may demonstrate alterations in awareness and movement caused by reaction to emotions. The initial difficulties with this phenomenon regards the name given to it. Table 9 lists some of the names used, which can be criticised for being too all encompassing (the term non-epileptic attack disorder [NEAD] would also describe migraine or syncope) or suggest deceit. While debates among medical professionals can often appear inflated, I have some sympathy with this one - getting over the nuance and implications of this syndrome is so important in shaping prognosis that the patient's reaction to the name will be critical. For brevity's sake, we will stick with pseudoseizure for this chapter, but you should be aware that patients may wrongly infer an epileptic basis, while doctors may wrongly infer insight and motivation from the patient.

Table 9 Naming non-epileptic attacks.

- Pseudoseizures

- Non-epileptic attacks

- Psychogenic non-epileptic seizures (PNES)

Frequency

Pseudoseizures are not rare; the frequency of this as a diagnosis at the first seizure clinic varies depending on the confidence of the doctor. Some estimates suggest that 4% of patients attending clinics have pseudoseizures. Many patients with syncopal attacks may well have some aggravation by anxiety - one man's 'syncope' is another man's pseudoseizure.

History

It is striking that so many patients with non-epileptic attacks will be unable to tell you about their attacks. A shrinking period of amnesia is usual among these patients, as prompting will help uncover more and more recall around individual events. Academic linguists have been able to demonstrate why doctors find history-taking from pseudoseizure patients a draining experience, as the story changes and requires elaboration.

In taking a background history, many patients with pseudoseizures will outline an early history of adverse life experience including abuse (sexual and physical) and emotional neglect. Encounters with other traumatic events may be a direct trigger, but it should be noted that those who have been through adverse life experience also have the right to develop epilepsy!

The pattern of events is often the first clue to the diagnosis of pseudoseizures, since these are more likely to 'burst onto the scene' at high frequency with a high level of intrusion. Provocation by certain circumstances or emotions will also help signal an emotional cause, but can occur with some anxious patients with epilepsy. The onset will often be gradual with evolving auditory or visual symptoms.

Eye witness history

Eye witnesses will help provide the background to the episodes, allowing contextualisation of the attacks. They will often be able to provide a good picture of the emotions and provocations surrounding each attack and the background to the onset of the disorder.

Description of the attack itself can also be most revealing with features that are strongly suggestive of pseudoseizures (see Table 10); attacks that are very prolonged, involving motor phenomena such as repetitive motor movements, absence of tone, pelvic thrusting, whole body rigidity, flailing or rhythmical co-ordinated movements, side to side head movements, and tremulous movements. Crying and upset on recovery is more frequent in patients after pseudoseizures.

Table 10 Features suggesting pseudoseizures.

Duration	Prolonged (hours)
Pattern	Very frequent at onset Provocation by events
Nature of attack	Thrusting Alternating movements Back arching
Associated features	Crying Anxious Hyperventilation

Diagnosis

Diagnosis is probably the crucial aspect of management of pseudoseizures, based on the combination of history and seizure observation. Once the diagnosis has been made and communicated properly this will help reduce attack frequency, leaving many patients free of episodes altogether. Even where this is the case, capturing an attack on EEG provides a useful tool for education and persuasion of the patient and family. Showing them that the EEG is unaffected during these episodes, and that there is no risk of cardiovascular or respiratory compromise is often a first step in convincing families and carers that hospitalisation and treatment of individual attacks is not necessary.

EEG with provocation and suggestion is a recognised way of providing hard evidence which, with video recording, can elicit information from both the patient and the family as to whether the recorded episode is typical. Use of this type of EEG protocol may avoid the use of resource-intensive longer-term inpatient monitoring.

Once the diagnosis has been confirmed (in both the doctor's and the patient's mind), then the process of treatment can begin, the initial moves often being to uncover other predisposing factors and contributory events that may not have become apparent during the initial assessments. At this stage, childhood events may become apparent.

Imaging

Where there is any doubt about the origin of attacks, then imaging is important to help allay any fears that the episodes are related to an intracranial lesion.

Management of NEAD

Definitive diagnosis is a vital step. It is vital to put the diagnosis of NEAD to the patient with the relevant care and preparation. Video evidence can prove vital in gaining trust and support from the family, particularly where they know that AED use will not help reduce or prevent attacks.

It is important that the patient should not be allowed to feel that psychological input is a second-best treatment or a sign that they are mad or malingering. Rather, it should be perceived as an empowerment; a way of helping the patient develop their own strategies and tactics.

Conclusions

Females with epilepsy should have some consideration taken as to how epilepsy and its treatment will affect their reproductive status, their exposure to hormonal supplements, and their risk of later complications such as osteoporosis.

The first job in a first seizure clinic is to find out who has fitted and who has fainted. Once the diagnosis of seizure is made, the patient should have reasonable investigations ordered, and be counselled about the risks of recurrence. For most patients, recurrence will not happen.

The management of seizures in patients with learning difficulties can at first seem a daunting experience. Setting achievable and realistic goals can help families and patients adjust to the onset of seizures. There is a lower chance of achieving seizure freedom, and assessment of efficacy and tolerability is more complex than in other patients. In fact, dealing with such patients and their families can be one of the most rewarding relationships, but only if all parties concerned are able to understand what goals are realisable and attainable.

Early diagnosis of pseudoseizures leads to better response rates, and less exposure to potentially hazardous medications. Clinical clues may make the diagnosis apparent, even long after anti-epileptic drugs have been started.

Key Summary

- One of the fascinating aspects of caring for patients with epilepsy is that you see patients in many different phases.

- Care of pregnant patients requires consideration of best treatment for them and their baby.

- Patients with learning difficulties present a range of challenges from over- to under-diagnosis of seizures.

- Diagnosis of pseudoseizures is important - it reduces exposure to inappropriate treatment and medical intervention.

- If in doubt about episodes, treat as seizures - it is less risky in the short term to over-treat than under-treat.

References

1. Marson A, Jacoby A, Johnson A, Kim L, Gamble C, Chadwick D. Immediate versus deferred antiepileptic drug treatment for early epilepsy and single seizures: a randomised controlled trial. *Lancet* 2005; 365: 2007-13.

Chapter 14
Common questions

Questions your patients will ask you

The aim of this chapter is to prepare you for some likely questions that your newly diagnosed patient will probably ask. Questions relating to women's issues and those of the elderly and children have been omitted; hopefully they have been covered in enough detail in earlier chapters. This is not an extensive list but aims to cover the most important topics that a newly diagnosed patient will have to face.

No questions at all!

This is the most worrying. Start with providing your patient with sources of information about epilepsy and contact information for local epilepsy support groups. Below are some useful websites with lots of information aimed at those with epilepsy:

- http://www.ibe-epilepsy.org/;
- http://www.epilepsyfoundation.org/;
- http://www.equip.nhs.uk/HealthTopics/epilepsy.aspx;
- www.epilepsyaction.org;
- www.epilepsyscotland.org.

Try to initiate the patient in a conversation, addressing their greatest concerns. It is also important to discuss some of the topics below, including driving, lifestyle changes and the importance of compliance.

Why do I have epilepsy?

For most adults, the exact cause of epilepsy is undiscovered, even after extensive investigation. We assume that many people with epilepsy have had a tiny area of scarring of the brain.

Will I have to tell my employer?

No-one should be putting themselves or other employees at risk if they have a seizure at work. The nature of any seizures and their frequency may need to be discussed with the occupational health department at your workplace. Many employees will be only too happy to be as accommodating as possible to allow employment to continue with minimum risk to the individual and their workmates.

Will I be able to drive?

Regulation of driving privileges varies greatly from country to country and state to state. Most regulatory authorities are not concerned with whether patients are on treatment, but only on how long patients have been seizure-free for a specified period of time.

This is a difficult subject to discuss with your patient. Often patients see driving as a right and not a privilege. Driving in many cases is not just a symbol of their independence but is also necessary for employment, caring for their family, etc. Often the loss of their driving licence evokes feelings of punishment and can lead to low self-esteem, cause social restrictions and lifestyle upsets, in addition to an increased dependability on others around them. It is important that you stress that the goal of these restrictions is to protect them and others. Acknowledge the frustration and inconvenience, note that the physician does not enforce these restrictions, the law does and also discuss the alternatives available to the patient.

As a physician, it is your responsibility to know the driving laws with regard to seizures in the area where you live. Regardless of your location, you are obligated to tell your patient about the dangers of driving and inform them of the appropriate restrictions. Some countries require you to report the diagnosis of epilepsy to the Department of Transportation. The seizure-free interval required from place to place varies greatly. In the USA it varies with state from 3 months to 2 years, in Europe some countries require a 2-year seizure-free interval, while others only require 1 year (e.g. UK). The European Union recommends an interval of 1-year seizure-freedom. It is important for legal liability that you, the physician, document this discussion; later, if a patient is in an accident the physician may be held at fault if there is no proof that the patient was warned.

Will I lose my job?

In most countries, an employer is not legally allowed to fire an employee because they have epilepsy. With this in mind, informing their employers should not jeopardize a patient's employment. Indeed, employers are often willing to accommodate the needs of the patient.

There are certain areas of employment that are not suitable for patients with epilepsy. Any job that the patient's sudden loss of consciousness would put themselves or others in danger is inappropriate, for example, anything involving heights, driving or the use of machinery.

Will I be on these drugs for life?

Many patients with epilepsy like to discuss coming off treatment after they have been seizure-free for a while. The chances of successfully coming off depends on a number of factors (duration of seizure freedom, presence of EEG changes, seizure type, and whether any seizures have been experienced on treatment), and the future chances of doing well on and off treatment should be discussed before the decision is made.

Are my epilepsy drugs addictive?

No.

Can I safely take the generic form of my drug instead?

European and U.S. authorities require every generic drug to be measurably similar to the original branded product. The danger with generic drugs is in frequent switches between generics and branded medications that may lead to subtle but important changes in blood levels and increase the risk of side effects and seizures. If a generic is to be used, it should always be the same make of generic.

I accidently missed a dose of my AED, should I wait until the next dose?

No. The dose should be taken as soon as you realize it has been missed. Missing a single dose should not cause problems. If, however, this is a regular occurrence it could lead to an insufficient concentration of the AED in the blood and lead to break-through seizures. If the patient reports missing a dose, preventative measures should be encouraged such as setting alarms on mobile phones or post-it notes which can help overcome this problem.

What about alternative medicine for the treatment of epilepsy?

There are no proper studies that have measured and compared the effectiveness of types of alternative medicine to AED treatment. Some herbal remedies may interfere with the metabolism of AEDs and a few (St John's wort, echinacea) are said to be associated with increased seizure tendency.

Is it safe to take multi-vitamin tablets?

Yes. Many of the AEDs can lead to deficiencies in thiamine, folic acid, magnesium, calcium and vitamin D. Indeed, a deficiency in vitamin B6 is known to be a cause of intractable seizures. Likewise, thiamine deficiency has also been associated with seizures. A daily multi-vitamin tablet is advisable for all patients with epilepsy, regardless of age or gender.

Do I have to avoid alcohol?

Advice to patients with epilepsy is exactly the same as for those with no epilepsy: moderation is no threat to health. Alcohol excess poses particular risk for patients with epilepsy, largely in its tendency to have more numerous and longer seizures (probably as a result of alcohol's effect in reducing depth of proper sleep). Alcohol in any amount should not prevent the patient from taking their medication - avoiding treatment because of worries about interactions will only further increase the likelihood of seizures.

What about street drugs?

Patients taking street drugs are at especially high risk of having seizures or worsening seizure control. Ecstasy, amphetamines, and cocaine are particularly prone to inducing more seizures. The effect of other drugs such as marijuana and heroin may be to induce a more chaotic lifestyle which may cause further worsening of seizure control. Don't forget that prescription-only medication such as benzodiazepines can induce seizures, if taken at inappropriate doses, inappropriate schedules, or withdrawn abruptly.

I'm having trouble with my memory, is there anything we can do about it?

Memory complaints are common in the epilepsy clinic. There are several reasons why this may be so. Some patients feel that AEDs may impair memory and concentration, so it is reasonable to ensure that patients are on the lowest doses of a minimum number of AEDs. Seizures themselves may hamper the brain's ability to store and retrieve information, so it is important to try and minimize seizure counts.

Mood difficulties are more common in people with epilepsy, and such disorders may present with perception of poor memory. Mood difficulties should not be allowed to develop into clinical depression.

I'm feeling down, do you think it is because of my medications?

Patients with epilepsy have an increased incidence of depression, with resultant changes in their appetite, motivation and sleep. Such mood problems may result from seizures, or the social effects of epilepsy. AEDs themselves will not usually cause depression.

Will the drugs affect any other treatments I am on?

Any doctor prescribing any other treatment should be aware that the patient is on anti-epileptic drugs so that they can make sure they do not interact. For most newer anti-epileptic drugs, the risk of significant interactions is low.

Will epilepsy stop me taking part in sports?

Some are more dangerous and not advisable. Swimming is advisable only when there is one-to-one supervision. Horseback-riding, gymnastics, ice-skating and bicycling are usually not suitable as loss of consciousness would usually involve trauma to the head. Likewise, competitive team sports involving contact (e.g. hockey, karate) or high impact (e.g. rugby, American football) are also risky as any brain injury may lead to the worsening of seizures. Parachuting, hang-gliding, climbing, scuba-diving are extremely dangerous and not advisable. Relatively non-contact sports such as football (soccer), basketball and volleyball are excellent team sports for people with seizure disorders, especially where coaches +/or team mates are aware of the condition. Track-and-field events are also suitable choices.

Will I be able to get pregnant?

Epilepsy itself does not prevent women from getting pregnant. Some drugs may change ovulation patterns and make becoming pregnant more difficult. For anyone on anti-epileptic drugs, pregnancy should be discussed with an epilepsy specialist beforehand; this will allow pre-planning of drug treatments and provision of folate supplements.

Will the drugs affect the development of my baby in the womb?

Among women with epilepsy, over 95% of pregnancies pass without complication. Some drugs are known to be associated with a slightly higher risk of developmental problems, and this is why it is helpful to have a discussion before the patient becomes pregnant to try and minimise the risks as much as possible.

Will I be able to breastfeed my baby when I'm on anti-epileptic drugs?

The baby will already have been exposed to the drugs for some months while the patient was pregnant. The concentration of the drug in the breastmilk will be low and not likely to cause any changes in the short or long-term health of the baby.

Is it safe for me to look after my children?

With simple measures, it is usually safe for all women with epilepsy to look after children even at a young age. Asking the question "would my baby be safe if I were to have a seizure here?" is as good a safety screen as any. Using this will often avoid situations such as bathing young children in deep water or letting them play in potentially hazardous environments.

Will my children get epilepsy too?

Children born to mothers with epilepsy have a slightly raised chance of inheriting the condition (approximately 2% higher than the background population risk). Fathers do not have a significant chance of passing on the condition.

What should I tell my friends to do when I have a seizure?

The first job is to make sure that the patient is removed from anything that may cause them harm during a seizure. Lying the patient in the recovery position will minimise the risk of injury and impairment of breathing. The vast majority of seizures will pass off without complication even if there is no-one to help.

Do my relatives need to call an ambulance every time I have a seizure?

By far the majority of seizures pass off without complication. The low risk of harm with shorter seizures means that medical assistance is more inconvenient then helpful! If seizures are prolonged (more than 5 minutes) or recur without recovering consciousness then emergency medical assistance should be sought.

Is there anything I can do to help prevent seizures?

As a general rule, taking medication regularly, avoiding excess alcohol intake, and having a good sleep pattern will help reduce seizures. Some people with epilepsy have noticed that specific factors will bring seizures on or make them more likely to happen.

Will seizures cause any further brain damage?

Prolonged seizures (so-called status epilepticus) can cause some brain cells to die, but this does not result in any change in function evident clinically. For the vast majority of seizures, there will be no effect.

Do I need to move house?

Receiving a diagnosis of epilepsy is bad enough without the need for dramatic changes in living arrangements. Some patients feel safer if they are not living alone, feeling that it reduces risk during seizures if someone is there to help. Absence of stairs may reduce risk of serious falls. There are many little changes that can make a household more 'seizure friendly'. Here is a short list:

Bathroom:

◆ showers have less risk of drowning than a bathtub;
◆ reducing risk of seizing unattended, by telling others they are going for a bath.

Kitchen:

◆ avoiding cooking while alone;
◆ use the back-burners on cookers/stoves preferably to reduce burns;
◆ keep the handles on saucepans facing inward;
◆ microwave cooking where possible;
◆ electric kettles should have an automatic switch off;
◆ tableware and cookware should be unbreakable if possible.

Other rooms:

◆ carpeting or rugs break impact of falls;
◆ forced-air heating is preferable to exposed heating elements, e.g. fan heaters, radiators;
◆ all fragile and breakable objects should be removed, including lamps and ornaments;
◆ reduce number of sharp edges on furniture.

Should video games be banned?

Patients with photosensitive epilepsy (PSE) should refrain from playing any video games, as they can provoke seizures easily. Indeed, there have been reports of patients with non-photosensitive epilepsy having seizures while playing video games. By law, all video-game manufacturers are required to put a clear warning for PSE and these games should be avoided by all patients with epilepsy. Similarly, video games should not encourage the patient to become sleep deprived. Other strategies to avoid the provocation of seizures include keeping an appropriate distance from the screen (2m), not playing while tired or playing continually for several hours.